CONTENTS

AN OPEN LETTER

DEVELOPMENT OF THE CHILD

FAULTS AND THEIR REMEDIES

CHARACTER BUILDING

PLAY

OCCUPATIONS

ART AND LITERATURE IN CHILD LIFE

STUDIES AND ACCOMPLISHMENTS

FINANCIAL TRAINING

RELIGIOUS TRAINING

APPLICATION OF PRINCIPLES

OTHER PEOPLE'S CHILDREN

THE SEX QUESTION

FATHERS

THE UNCONSCIOUS INFLUENCE

ANSWERS TO QUESTIONS

BIBLIOGRAPHY

SUPPLEMENTAL STUDY PROGRAM

INDEX

AMERICAN SCHOOL OF HOME ECONOMICS
CHICAGO

January 1, 1907.

My dear Madam:

In beginning this subject of the "Study of Child Life" there may be lurking doubts in your mind as to whether any reliable rules can really be laid down. They seem to arise mostly from the perception of the great difference between children. What will do for one child will not do for another. Some children are easily persuaded and gentle, others willful, still others sullen unresponsive. How, then, is it possible that a system of education and training can be devised suitable for their various dispositions?

We must remember that children are much more alike than they are different. One may have blue eyes, another gray, another black, but they all have two. We are, therefore, in a position to make rules for creatures having two eyes and these rules apply to eyes of all colors. Children may be nervous, sanguine, bilious, or plethoric, but they all have the same kind of internal organs end the same general rules of health apply to them all.

In this series of lessons I have endeavored to set forth principles briefly and to confirm them by instances within the experience of every observer of childhood. The rules given are such as are held at present by the best educators to be based upon sound philosophy, not at variance with the slight array or scientific facts at our command. Perhaps you yourself may be able to add to the number of reliable facts intelligently reported that must be collected before much greater scientific advance is possible.

There is, to be sure, an art of application of these rules both in matters of health of body and of health of mind and this art must be worked out by each mother for each individual child.

We all recognize that it is a long endeavor before we can apply to our own lives such principles of conduct as we heartily acknowledge to be right. Why, then, expect to be able to apply principles instantly and unerringly to a little child? If a rule fails when you attempt to apply it, before questioning the principle, may it not be well to question your own tact and skill?

So far as I can advise with you in special instances of difficulty, I shall be very glad to do so; not that I shall always know what to do myself, but that we can get a little more light upon the problems by conferring together. I know well how difficult a matter this of child training is, for every day, in the management of my own family of children, I find each philosophy, science and art as I can command very much put to the test.

Sincerely yours,

Marion Foster Washburne,

    Instructor

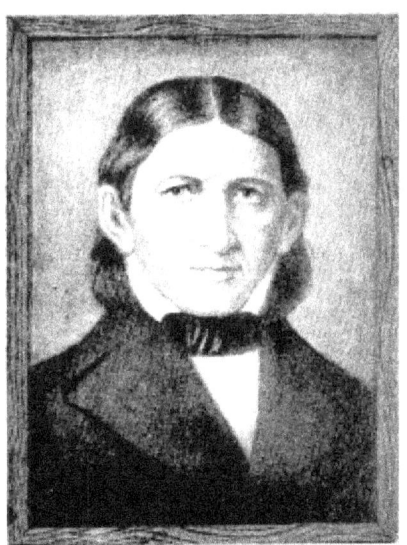

FRIEDRICH FROEBEL.
By courtesy of The Perry Pictures Co. Malden, Mass.

STUDY OF CHILD LIFE

PART I.

The young of the human species is less able to care for itself than the young of any other species. Most other creatures are able to walk, or at any rate stand, within a few hours of birth. But the human baby is absolutely dependent and helpless, unable even to manufacture all the animal heat that he requires. The study of his condition at birth at once suggests a number of practical procedures, some of them quite at variance with the traditional procedures.

HOW THE CHILD DEVELOPS

Condition at Birth

Let us see, then, exactly what his condition is. In the first place, he is, as Virchow, an authority on physiological subjects declares, merely a spinal animal. Some of the higher brain centers do not yet exist at all, while others are in too incomplete a state for service. The various sensations which the baby experiences—heat, light, contact, motion, etc.—are so many stimuli to the development of these centers. If the stimulus is too great, the development is sometimes unduly hastened, with serious results, which show themselves chiefly in later life. The child who is brought up a noisy room, is constantly talked to and fondled, is likely to develop prematurely, to talk and walk at an early age; also to fall into nervous decay at an early age. And even if by reason of an unusually good heredity he escapes these dangers, it is almost certain that his intellectual power is not so great in adult life as it would have been under more favorable conditions. A new baby, like a young plant, requires darkness and quiet for the most part. As he grows older, and shows a spontaneous interest in his surroundings, he may fittingly have more light, more companionship, and experience more sensations.

Weight at Birth

The average boy baby weighs about seven pounds at birth; the average girl, about six and a half pounds. The head is larger in proportion to the body than in after life; the nose is incomplete, the legs short and bowed, with a tendency to fall back upon the body with the knees flexed. This natural tendency should be allowed full play, for the flexed position is said to be favorable to the growth of the bones, permitting the cartilaginous ends of the bones to lie free from pressure at the joints.

The plates of the skull are not complete and do not fit together at the edges. Great care needs to be taken of the soft spot thus left exposed on the top of the head—the undeveloped place where the edges of these bones come together. Any injury here in early life is liable to affect the mind.

State of Development

The bony enclosures of the middle ear are unfinished and the eyes also are unfinished. It is a question yet to be settled, whether a new-born baby is blind and deaf or not. At a rate, he soon acquires a sensitiveness to both light and sound, although it is three years or more before he has amassed sufficient experience to estimate with accuracy the distance of objects seen or herd. He can cry, suck, sneeze, cough, kick, and hold on to a finger. All of these acts, though they do not yet imply personality, or even mind, give evidence of a wonderful organism. They require the co-operation of many delicate nerves and muscles—a co-operation that has as yet baffled the power of scientists to explain.

Although the young baby is in almost constant motion while he is awake, he is altogether too weak to turn himself in bed or to escape from an uncomfortable position, and he remains so for many weeks. This constant motion is necessary to his muscular development, his control of his own muscles, his circulation, and, very probably, to the free transmission of nervous energy. Therefore, it is of the first importance that he has freedom to move, and he should be given time every day to move and stretch before the fire, without clothes on. It is well to rub his back and legs at the same time, thus supplementing his gymnastics with a gentle massage.

Educational Beginnings.

By the time he is four or five weeks old it is safe to play with him, a little every day, and Froebel has made his "Play with the Limbs" one of his first educational exercises. In this play the mother lays the baby, undressed, upon a pillow and catches the little ankles in her hands. Sometimes she prevents the baby from kicking, so that he has to struggle to get his legs free; sometimes she helps him, so that he kicks more freely and regularly; sometimes she lets him push hard against her breast. All the time she laughs and sings to him, and Froebel has made a little song for this purposes. Since consciousness is roused and deepened by sensations, remembered, experienced, and compared, it is evident that this is more than a fanciful play; that it is what Froebel claimed for it—a real educational exercise. By means, of it the child may gain some consciousness of companionship, and thus, by contrast, a deeper self-consciousness.

First Efforts

The baby is at first unable to hold up its head, and in this he is just like all other animals, for no animal, except man, holds up its head constantly. The human baby apparently makes the effort, because he desires to see more clearly—he could doubtless see clearly enough for all physical purposes with his head hung down, but not enough to satisfy his awakening mentality. The effort to hold the head up and to look around is therefore regarded by most psychologists as one of the first tokens of an awakening intellectual life. And this is true, although the first effort seems to arise from an overplus of nervous energy which makes the neck muscles contract, just as it makes other muscles contract. The first slight raisings of the head are like the first kicking movements, merely impulsive; but the child soon sees the advantage of this apparently accidental movement and tries to master it. Preyer [A] considers that the efforts to balance the head among the first indications that the child's will is taking possession of his muscles. His own boy arrived at this point when he was between three and four months old.

Reflex Grasping

The grasp of the new-born baby's hand has a surprising power, but the baby himself has little to do with it. The muscles act because of a stimulus presented by the touch of the fingers, very much as the muscles of a decapitated frog contract when the current of electricity passes over them. This is called reflex grasping, and Dr. Louis Robinson, [B] thinking that this early strength of gasp was an important illustration of and evidence for evolution, tried experiments on some sixty new-born babies. He found that they could sustain their whole weight by the arms alone when their hands were clasped about a slender rod. They grasped the rod at once and could be lifted from the bed by it and kept in this position about half a minute. He argued that this early strength of arm, which soon begins to disappear, was survival from the remote period when the baby's ancestors were monkeys or monkey-like people who lived in trees.

Beginnings Of Will Power

However this may be, during the first week the baby's hands are much about his face. By accident they reach, the mouth, they are sucked; the child feels himself suck its own fist; he feels his fist being sucked. Some day it will occur to him that that fist belongs to the same being who owns the sucking mouth. But at this point, Miss Shinn[C] has observed, the baby is often surprised and indignant that he cannot move his arms around and at the same time suck his fist. This discomfort helps him to make an effort to get his fist into his mouth and keep it there, and this effort shows his will, beginning to take possession of his hands and arms.

Growth of Will

Since any faculty grows by its own exercise, just as muscles grow by exercise, every time the baby succeeds in getting his hands to his mouth as a result of desire, every time that he succeeds in grasping an object as result of desire, his will power grows. Action of this nature brings in new sensations, and the brain centers used for recording such sensations grow.

As the sensations multiply, he compares them, and an idea is born. For the beginnings of mental development no other mechanism is actually needed than a brain and a hand and the nerves connecting them. Laura Bridgeman and Helen Keller, both of them deaf and blind, received their education almost entirely through their hands, and yet they were unusually capable of thinking. The child's hands, then, from the beginning, are the servants of his brain-instruments by means of which he carries impressions from the outer world to the seat of consciousness, and by which in turn he imprints his consciousness upon the outer world.

Intentional Grasping

The average baby does not begin to grasp objects with intention before the fourth month. The first grasping seems to be done by feeling, without the aid of the eye, and is done with the fingers with no attempt to oppose the thumb to them. So closely does the use of the thumbs set opposite the fingers in grasping coincide with the first grasping with the aid of sight, that some observers have been led to believe that as soon as the baby learns to use its thumb in this way he proves that he is beginning to grasp with intention.

Order of Development

The order of development seems to be, *first*, automatism, the muscles contracting of themselves in response to nervous stimuli; *second*, instinct, the inherited wisdom of the race, which discovered ages ago that the hand could be used to greater advantage when the thumb was separated from the fingers; and *thirdly,* the child's own intelligence and will making use of this natural and inherited machinery. This order holds true of the development, not only of the hand, but of the whole organism.

Looking

A little earlier than this, during the third month, the baby first looks upon his own hands and notices them. Darwin tells us that his boy looked at his own hands and seemed to study them until his eyes crossed. About the same then the child notices his foot and uses his hand to carry it to its mouth. It is some time later that he discovers that he can move his feet without his hands.

Tearing

About this time, three or four months old, the child begins to tear paper into pieces, and may be easily taught to let the piece, that have found their way into his mouth be taken out again. Now, too, he begins to throw things, or to drop them; then he wants to get them back again, and the patient mother must pick them up and give them back many times. Sometimes a baby is punished for this proclivity, but it is really a part of his development, and at least once a day he should be allowed to play in this manner to his heart's content. It is tact, not discipline, that is needed, and the more he is helped the sooner he will live through this stage and come to the next point where he begins to throw things.

Throwing

In this stage, of course, he must be given the proper things to throw—small, bright-colored worsted balls, bean-bags, and other harmless objects. If he is allowed to discover the pleasure there is in smashing glass and china, he will certainly be, for a time, a very destructive little person. When later he is able to creep throw his ball and creep after it—he will amuse himself for hours at a time, and so relieve those who have patiently attended him up to this time. *In general we may lay down the rule, that the more time and attention of the right sort is to a young child, the less will need to be given as he grows older.* It is poor economy to neglect a young child, and try to make it up on the growing boy or girl. This is to substitute a complicated and difficult problem for a simple one.

The Grasping Instinct

It is some time before a child's will can so overcome his newly-acquired tendency to grasp every possible object that he can keep his hand off of anything that invites him. The many battles between mothers and children it the subject of not touching forbidden things are at this stage a genuine wrong and injustice to the child. So young a child is scarcely more responsible for touching whatever he can reach that is a piece of steel for being drawn toward a powerful magnet. Preyer says that it is years before voluntary inhibitions of grasping become possible. The child has not the necessary brain machinery. Commands and sparring of the hands create bewilderment and tend to build up a barrier between mother and child. Instead of doing such thing, simply put high out of reach and sight whatever the child must not touch.

Another way in which young children are often made to suffer because of the ignorance of parents is the leaving of undesired food on the child's plate. Every child, when he does not want his food, pushes the plate away from him, and many mothers push it back and scold. The real truth is that the motor suggestion of the food upon the plate is so strong that the child feels as if he were being forced to eat it every time he looks at the plate; to escape from eating it he is obliged to push it out of sight.

The Three Months' Baby

But this difficulty comes later. Now we are concerned with a three-months-old baby. At this stage the child is usually able to balance his head, to sit up against pillows, to seize and grasp objects, and to hold out his arm, when he wishes to be taken. Although he may have made number of efforts to sit erect, and may have succeeded for a few minutes at a time, he still is far from being able to sit alone, unsupported. This he does not accomplish until the fifth or the month.

Danger of Forcing

There is nothing to be gained by trying to make him sit alone sooner; indeed, there is danger in it—danger in forcing young bones and muscles to do work beyond their strength, and danger also to the nerves. It is safe to say that *a normal child always exercises all its faculties to the utmost without need of urging, and any exercise beyond the point of natural fatigue, if persisted in, is sure to bring about abnormal results.*

Creeping

The first efforts toward creeping often appear in the bath when the child turns over and raise, himself upon his hands and knees. This is sign that he might creep sooner, if he were not impeded by clothing. He should be allowed to spread himself upon a blanket every day for an hour or two, and to get on his knees as frequently as he pleases. Often he needs a little help to make him creep forward, for most babies creep backward at first, their arms being stronger than their legs. Here the mother may safely interfere, pushing the legs as they ought to go and showing the child how to manage himself; for very often he becomes much excited over his inability to creep forward.

The climbing instinct begins to appear by this time—the seventh month—and here the stair-case has its great advantages. It ought not to be shut from him by a gate, but he should be taught how to climb up and down it in safety. To do this, start him at the head of the stairs, and, you yourself being below him, draw first one knee and then the other over the step, thus showing him how to creep backward. Two lessons of about twenty minutes each will be sufficient. The only danger is creeping down head foremost, but if he once learns thoroughly to go backward, and has not been allowed the other way at all, he will never dream of trying it. In going down backward, if he should slip, he can easily save himself by catching the stairs with his hands as he slips past.

The child who creeps is often later in his attempts to walk than the child who does not; and, therefore, when he is ready to walk, his legs will be all the stronger, and the danger of bow-legs will be past. As long as the child remains satisfied with creeping, he is not yet ready either mentally or physically for walking.

Standing

If the child has been allowed to creep about freely, he will soon be standing. He will pull himself to his feet by means of any chair, table, or indeed anything that he may get hold of. To avoid injuring him, no flimsy chairs or spindle-legged tables should be allowed in his nursery. He will next begin to sidle around a chair, shuffling his feet in a vague fashion, and sometimes, needing both of his hands to seize some coveted object, he will stand without clinging, leaning on his stomach. An unhurried child may remain at this stage for weeks.

Walking

Let alone, as he should be, he will walk without knowing how he does it, and will be the stronger for having overcome his difficulties himself. He should not be coaxed to stand or walk. The things in his room actually urge him to come and get them. Any further persuasion is forced, and may urge him beyond his strength.

Walking-chairs and baby-jumpers are injurious in this respect. They keep the child from his native freedom of sprawling, climbing, and pulling himself up. The activity they do permit is less varied and helpful than the normal activity, and the child, restricted from the preparatory motions, begins to walk too soon.

Alternate Growth

A curious fact in the growth of children is that they seem to grow heavier for a certain period, and then to grow taller for a similar period. That is, a very young baby, say, two months old, will grow fatter for about six weeks, and then for the next six weeks will grow longer, while the child of six years changes his manner of growth every three or four months. These periods are variable, or at least their law has not yet been established, but the observant mother can soon make the period out for herself in the case of her own child. For two or three days, when the manner of growth seems to be changing from breadth to length, and vice versa, the children are likely to be unusually nervous and irritable, and these aberrations must, of course, be patiently borne with.

Precocity

Early Ripening

In all these things some children develop earlier than others, but too early development is to be regretted. Precocious children are always of a delicate nervous organization. Fiske [D] has proved to us that the reason why the human young is so far more helpless and dependent than the young of any other species is because the activities of the human race have become so many, so widely varied, and so complex, that they could not fix themselves in the nervous structure before birth. There a only a few things that the chick needs to know in order to lead a successful chicken life; as a consequence these few things are well impressed upon the small brain before ever he chips the shell; but the baby needs to learn a great many things—so many that there is no time or room to implant them before birth, or indeed, in the few years immediately succeeding birth. To hurry the development, therefore, of certain few of these faculties, like the faculties of talking, and walking, of imitation or response, is to crowd out many other faculties perhaps just beginning to grow. Such forcing will limit the child's future development to the few faculties whose growth is thus early stimulated. Precocity in a child, therefore, is a thing to be deplored. His early ripening foretells a early decay and a wise mother is she who gives her child ample opportunity for growing, but no urging.

Ample Opportunity for Growth

Ample opportunity for growth includes (1) Wholesome surroundings, (2) Sufficient sleep, (3) Proper clothing, (4) Nourishing food. We will take up these topics in order.

[A]

    W. Preyer. Professor of Physiology, of Jena, author of "The Mind of the Child." D. Appleton & Co.

[B]

    Dr. Robinson. Physician and Evolutionist, paper in The Eclectic, Vol. 29.

[C]

    Miss Millicent Shinn, American Psychologist, author of "Biography of a Baby."

[D]

John Fiske, writer on Evolutionary Philosophy. His theory of infancy is perhaps his most important contribution to science.

WHOLESOME SURROUNDINGS

The whole house in which the child lives ought to be well warmed and equally well aired. Sunlight also is necessary to his well-being. If it is impossible to have this in every room, as sometimes happens in city homes, at least the nursery must have it. In the central States of the Union plants and trees exposed to the southern sun put forth their leaves two weeks sooner than those exposed to the north. The infant cannot fail to profit by the same condition, for the young child may be said to lead in part a vegetative as well as an animal life, and to need air and sunshine and warmth as much as plants do. The very best room in the house is not too good for the nursery, for in no other room is such important and delicate work being done.

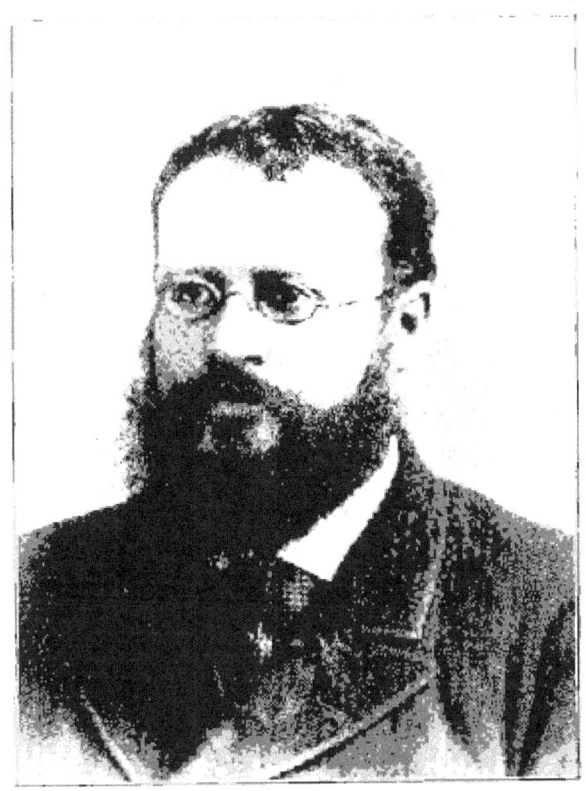

JOHN FISKE

Temperature

The temperature is a matter of importance. It should not be decided by guess-work, but a thermometer should be hung upon a wall at a place equally removed from draft and from the source of heat. The temperature for children during the first year should be about 70 degrees Fahrenheit during the day and not lower than 50 degrees at night. Children who sleep with the mother will not be injured by a temperature 5 to 20 degrees lower at night.

Fresh Air

It is important to provide means for the ingress of fresh air. It is not sufficient to air the room from another room unless that other room has in it an open window. Even then the nursery windows should be opened wide from fifteen minutes to half an hour night and morning, while the child is in another room; and this even when the weather is at zero or below. It does not take long to warm up room that has been aired. Perhaps the best means of obtaining the ingress of fresh air without creating a draft upon the floor, where the baby spends so much of his time, is to raise the window six inches at the top or bottom and insert a board cut to fit the aperture.

Daily Outing

But no matter how well ventilated the nursery may be, all children more than six weeks old need unmodified outside air, and need it every day, no matter what the weather, unless they are sick.

The daily outing secures them better appetites, quiet sleep, and calmer nerves. Let them be properly clothed and protected in their carriages, and all weathers are good for them.

Children who take their naps in their baby-carriages may with advantage be wheeled into a sheltered spot, covered warmly, and left to sleep in the outer air. They are likely to sleep longer than in the house, and find more refreshment in their sleep.

SUFFICIENT SLEEP.

Few children in America get as much sleep as they really need. Preyer gives the record of his own child, and the hours which this child found necessary for his sleep and growth may be taken for a standard. In the first month, sixteen, in full, out of twenty-four hours were spent in sleep. The sleep rarely lasted beyond two hours at a time. In the second month about the same amount was spent in sleep, which lasted from three to six hours at a time. In the sixth month, it lasted from six to eight hours at a time, and began to diminish to fifteen hours in the twenty-four. In the thirteenth month, fourteen hours' sleep daily; it the seventeenth, prolonged sleep began, ten hours without interruption; in the twentieth, prolonged sleep became habitual, and sleep in the day-time was reduced to two hours. In the third year, the night sleep lasted regularly from eleven to twelve hours, and sleep in the daytime was no longer required.

Naps

Preyer's record stops here. But it may be added that children from three to eight years still require eleven hours' sleep; and, although the child of three nay not need a daily nap, it is well for him, until he is six years old, to lie still for an hour in the middle of the day, amusing himself with a picture book or paper and pencil, but not played with or talked to by any other person. Such a rest in the middle of the day favors the relaxation of muscles and nerves and breaks the strain of a long day of intense activity.

PROPER CLOTHING.

Proper clothing for a child includes three things: (a) Equal distribution of warmth, (b) Freedom from restraint, (c) Light weight.

Equal distribution of warmth is of great importance, and is seldom attained. The ordinary dress for a young baby, for example, leaves the arms and the upper part of the chest unprotected by more than one thickness of flannel and one of cotton—the shirt and the dress. About the child's middle, on the contrary, there are two thicknesses of flannel—a shirt and band—and five of cotton, i.e., the double bands of the white and flannel petticoats, and the dress. Over the legs, again, are two thicknesses of flannel and two of cotton, i.e., the pinning blanket, flannel skirt, white skirt, and dress. The child in a comfortably warm house needs two thicknesses of flannel and one of cotton all over it, and no more.

The Gertrude Suit

The practice of putting extra wrappings about the abdomen is responsible for undue tenderness of those organs. Dr. Grosvenor, of Chicago, who designed a model costume for a baby, which he called the Gertrude suit, says that many cases of rupture are due to bandaging of the abdomen. When the child cries the abdominal walls normally expand; if they are tightly bound, they cannot do this, and the pressure upon one single part, which the bandages may not hold quite firmly, becomes overwhelming, and results in rupture. Dr. Grosvenor also thinks that many cases of weak lungs, and even of consumption in later life, are due to the tight bands of the skirts pressing upon the soft ribs of the young child, and narrowing the lung space.

Objection to the Pinning Blanket

Freedom from restraint.. Not only should the clothes not bind the child's body in any way, but they should not be so long as to prevent free exercise of the legs. The pinning-blanket is objectionable on this account. It is difficult for the child to kick in it; and as we have seen before, kicking is necessary to the proper development of the legs. Undue length of skirt operates in the same way—the weight of cloth is a check upon activity. The first garment of a young baby should not be more than a yard in length from the neck to the bottom of the hem, and three-quarters of a yard is enough for the inner garment.

The sleeves, too, should be large and loose, and the arm-size should be roomy, so as to prevent chafing. The sleeves may be tied in at the wrist with a ribbon to insure warmth.

Lightness of weight. The underclothing should be made of pure wool, so as to gain the greatest amount of warmth from the least weight. In the few cases where wool would cause irritation, a silk and wool fixture makes a softer but more expensive garment. Under the best conditions, clothes restrict and impede free development somewhat, and the heavier they are the more they impede it. Therefore, the effort should be to get the greatest amount of warmth with the least possible weight. Knit garments attain this most perfectly, but the next best thing is all-wool flannel of a fine grade. The weave known as stockinet is best of all, because goods thus made cling to the body and yet restrict its activity very little.

The best garments for a baby are made according to the accompanying diagram.

Princess Garment

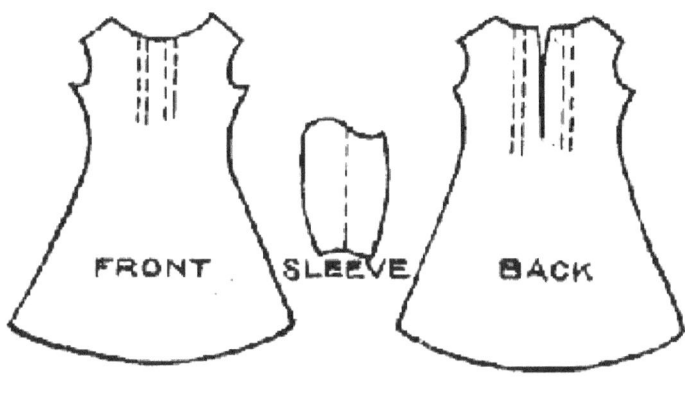

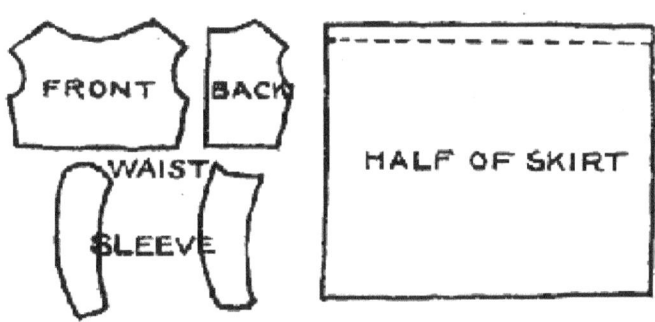

DIAGRAM OF THE "GERTRUDE" SUIT.

They consist of three garments, to be worn one over the other, each one an inch longer in every way than the underlying one. The first is a princess garment, made of white stockinet, which takes the place of shirt, pinning-blanket, and band. Before cutting this out, a box-pleat an inch and a half wide should be laid down the middle of the front, and a side pleat three-fourths of an inch wide on either side of the placket in the back. The sleeve should have a tuck an inch wide. These tucks and pleats are better run in be hand, so that they may be easily ripped. As the baby grows and the flannel shrinks, these tucks and pleats can be let out.

The next garment, which goes over this, is made in the same way, only an inch larger in every measurement. It is made of baby flannel, and takes the place of the flannel petticoat with its cotton band. Over these two garments any ordinary dress may be worn. Dressed in this suit, the child is evenly covered with too thicknesses of flannel and one of cotton. As the skirts are rather short, however, and he is expected to move his legs about freely, he may well wear long white wool stockings.

As the child grows older, the principles underlying this method of clothing should be borne in mind, and clothes should be designed and adapted so as to meet these three requirements.

FOOD.

Natural Food

Bottle-fed Babies

The natural food of a young baby is his mother's milk, and no satisfactory substitute for it has yet been found. Some manufactured baby foods do well for certain children; to others they are almost poison; and for none of them are they sufficient. The milk of the cow is not designed for the human infant. It contains too much casein, and is too difficult of digestion. Various preparations of milk and grains are recommended by nurses and physicians, but no conscientious nurse or physician pretends that any of them begins to equal the nutritive value of human milk. More women can nurse their babies than now think they can; the advertisements of patent foods lead them to think the rather of little importance, and they do not make the necessary effort to preserve and increase the natural supply of milk. The family physician can almost always better the condition of the mother who really desires to nurse her own child, and he should be consulted and his directions obeyed. The importance of a really great effort to this direction is shown by the fact that the physical culture records, now so carefully kept in many of our schools and colleges, prove that bottle-fed babies are more likely to be of small stature, and to have deficient bones, teeth and hair, than children who have been fed on mother's milk.

Simple Diet

The food question is undoubtedly the most important problem to the physical welfare of the child, and has, as well, a most profound effect upon his disposition and character. Indiscriminate feeding is the cause of much of the trouble and worry of mothers. This subject is taken up at length in other papers of this course, and it will suffice to say here that the table of the family with young children should be regulated largely by the needs of the growing sons and daughters. The simplified diet necessary may well be of benefit to other members of the family.

FAULTS AND THEIR REMEDIES.

The child born of perfect parents, brought up perfectly, in a perfect environment, would probably have no faults. Even such a child, however, would be at times inconvenient, and would do and say things at variance with the order of the adult world. Therefore he might seem to a hasty, prejudiced observer to be naughty. And, indeed, imperfectly born, imperfectly trained as children now are, many of their so-called faults are no more than such inconvenient crossings of an immature will with an adult will.

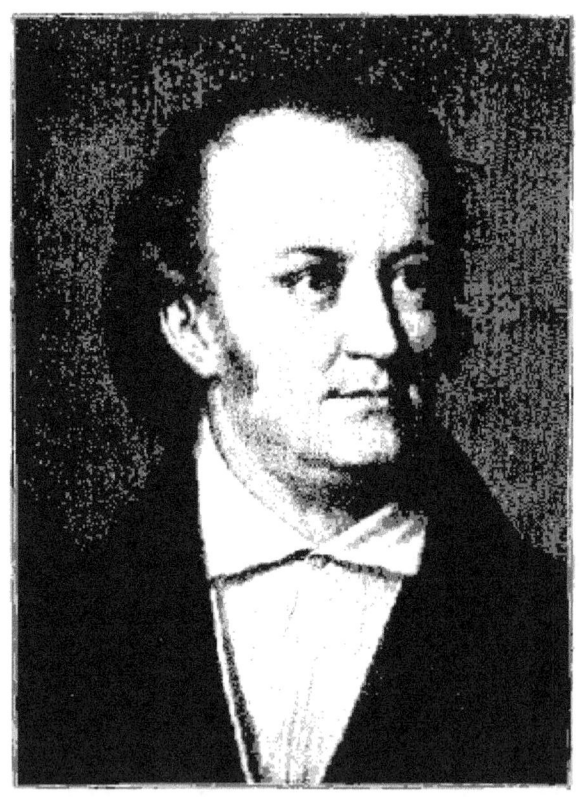

JEAN PAUL RICHTER

The Child's World and the Adult's World

No grown person, for instance, likes to be interrupted, and is likely to regard the child who interrupts him wilfully naughty. No young child, on the contrary, objects to being interrupted in his speech, though he may object to being interrupted in his play; and he cannot understand why an adult should set so much store on the quiet listening which is so infrequent in his own experience. Grown persons object to noise; children delight in it. Grown persons like to have things kept in their places; to a child, one place as good as another. Grown persons have a prejudice in favor of cleanliness; children like to swim, but hate to wash, and have no objections whatever to grimy hands and faces. None of these things imply the least degree of obliquity on the child's part; and yet it is safe to say that nine-tenths of the children who are punished are punished for some of these things. The remedy for these inconveniences is time and patience. The child, if left to himself, without a word of admonishment, would probably change his conduct in these respects, merely by the force of imitation, provided that the adults around him set him, a persistent example of courtesy, gentleness, and cleanliness.

Real Faults

The faults that are real faults, as Richter[A] says, are those faults which increase with age. These it is that need attention rather than those that disappear of themselves as the child grows older. This rule ought to be put in large letters, that every one who has to train children may be daily reminded by it; and not exercise his soul and spend his force in trying to overcome little things which may perhaps be objectionable, but which will vanish to-morrow. Concentrate your energies on the overcoming of such tendencies as may in time develop into permanent evils.

Training the Will

To accomplish this, you most, of course, train the child's own will, because no one can force another person into virtue against his will. The chief object of all training is, as we shall see in the next section, to lead the child to love righteousness, to prefer right doing to wrong doing; to make right doing a permanent desire. Therefore, in all the procedures about to be suggested, an effort is made to convince the child of the ugliness and painfulness of wrong doing.

Natural Punishment

Punishment, as Herbert Spencer [B] agrees with Froebel[C] in pointing out, should be as nearly as possible a representation of the natural result of the child's action; that is, the fault should be made to punish itself as much as possible without the interference of any outside person; for the object is not to make the child bend his will to the will of another, but make him see the fault itself as an undesirable thing.

Breaking the Will

The effort to break the child's will has long been recognized as disastrous by all educators. A broken will is worse misfortune than a broken back. In the latter case the man is physically crippled; in the former, he is morally crippled. It is only a strong, unbroken, persistent will that is adequate to achieve self-mastery, and mastery of the difficulties of life. The child who is too yielding and obedient in his early days is only too likely to be weak and incompetent in his later days. The habit of submission to a more mature judgment is a bad habit to insist upon. The child should be encouraged to think out things for himself; to experiment and discover for himself why his ideas do not work; and to refuse to give them up until he is genuinely convinced of their impracticability.

Emergencies

It is true that there are emergencies in which his immature judgment and undisciplined will must yield to wiser judgment and steadier will; but such yielding should not be suffered to become habitual. It is a safety valve merely, to be employed only when the pressure of circumstances threatens to become dangerous. An engine whose safety valve should be always in operation could never generate much power. Nor is there much difficulty in leading even a very strong-willed and obstinate child to give up his own way under extraordinary circumstances. If he is not in the habit of setting up his own will against that of his mother or teacher, he will not set it up when the quick, unfamiliar word of command seems to fit in the with the unusual circumstances. Many parents practice crying "Wolf! wolf!" to their children, and call the practice a drill of self-control; but they meet inevitably with the familiar consequences: when the real wolf comes the hackneyed cry, often proved false, is disregarded.

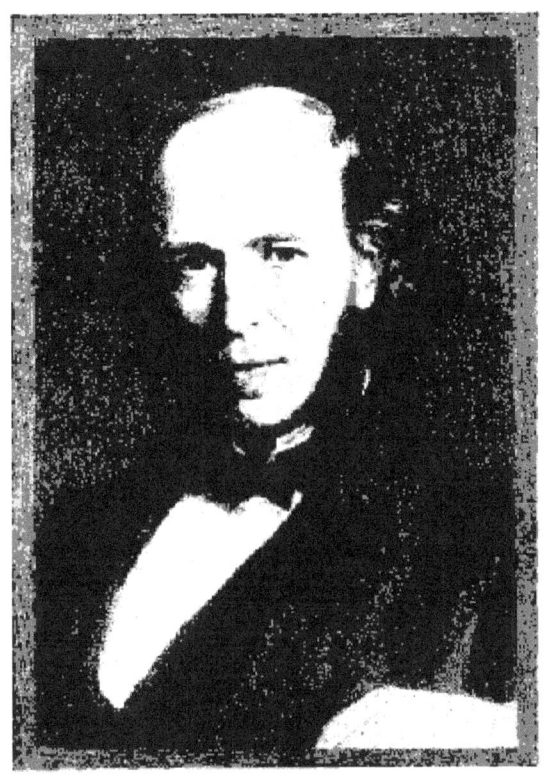

HERBERT SPENCER

Disobedience

When the will is rightly trained, disobedience is a fault that rarely appears, because, of course, where obedience is seldom required, it is seldom refused. The child needs to obey—that is true; but so does his mother need to obey, and all other persons about him. They all need to obey God, to obey the laws of nature, the impulses of kindness, and to follow after the ways of wisdom. Where such obedience is a settled habit of the entire household, it easily, and, as it were, unconsciously, becomes the habit of the child. Where such obedience is not the habit of the household, it is only with great difficulty that it can become the habit of the child. His will must set itself against its instinct of imitativeness, and his small house, not yet quite built, must be divided against itself. Probably no cold even rendered entire obedience to any adult who did not himself hold his own wishes in subjection. As Emerson says, "In dealing with my child, my Latin and my Greek, my accomplishments and my money, stead me nothing, but as much soul as I have avails. If I a willful, he sets his will against mine, one for one, and leaves me, if I please, the degradation of beating him by my superiority of strength. But, if I renounce my will and act for the soul, setting that up as an umpire between us two, out of his young eyes looks the same soul; he reveres and loves with me."

Negative Goodness

Suppose the child to be brought to such a stage that he is willing to do anything his father or mother says; suppose, even, that they never tell him to do anything that he does not afterwards discover to be reasonable and just; still, what has he gained? For twenty years he has not had the responsibility for a single action, for a single decision, right or wrong. What is permitted is right to him; what is forbidden is wrong. When he goes out into the world without his parents, what will happen? At the best he will not lie, or steal, or commit murder. That is, he will do none of these things in their bald and simple form.

But in their beginnings these are hidden under a mask of virtue and he has never been trained to look beneath that mask; as happened to Richard Feveril, [D] sin may spring upon him unaware. Some one else, all his life, has labeled things for him; he is not in the habit of judging for himself. He is blind, deaf, and helpless—a plaything of circumstances. It is a chance whether he falls into sin or remains blameless.

Real Disobedience

Disobedience, then, in a true sense, does not mean failure to do as he is told to do. It means failure to do the things that he knows to be right. He must be taught to listen and obey the voice of his own conscience; and if that voice should ever speak, as it sometimes does, differently from the voice of the conscience of his parents or teachers, its dictates must still be respected by these older and wiser persons, and he must be permitted to do this thing which in itself may be foolish, but which is not foolish, to him.

Liberty

And, on the other hand, the child who will have his own way even when he knows it to be wrong should be allowed to have it within reasonable limits. Richter says, leave to him the sorry victory, only exercising sufficient ingenuity to make sure that it is a sorry one. What he must be taught is that it is not at all a pleasure to have his own way, unless his own way happens to be right; and this he can only be taught by having his own way when the results are plainly disastrous. Every time that a willful child does what he wants to do, and suffers sharply for it, he learns a lesson that nothing but this experience can teach him.

Self-Punishment

But his suffering must be plainly seen to be the result of his deed, and not the result of his mother's anger. For example, a very young child who is determined to play with fire may be allowed to touch the hot lamp or a stove, whenever affairs can be so arranged that he is not likely to burn himself too severely. One such lesson is worth all the hand-spattings and cries of "No, no!" ever resorted to by anxious parents. If he pulls down the blocks that you have built up for him, they should stay down, while you get out of the room, if possible, in order to evade all responsibility for that unpleasant result.

Prohibitions are almost useless. In order to convince yourself of this, get some one to command you not to move your right arm or to wink your eye. You will find it almost impossible to obey for even a few moments. The desire to move your arm, which was not at all conscious before, will become overpowering. The prohibition acts like a suggestion, and is an implication that you would do the negative act unless you were commanded not to. Miss Alcott, in "Little Men," well illustrates this fact in the story of the children who were told not to put beans up their noses and who straightway filled their noses with beans.

Positive Commands

As we shall see in the next section, Froebel meets this difficulty by substituting positive commands for prohibitions; that is, he tells the child to do instead of telling him not to do. Tiedemann [E] says that example is the first great evolutionary teacher, and liberty is the second. In the overcoming of disobedience, no other teachers are needed. The method may be tedious; it may be many years before the erratic will is finally led to work in orderly channels; but there is no possibility of abridging the process. There is no short and sudden cure for disobedience, and the only hope for final cure is the steady working of these two great forces, *example* and *liberty*.

To illustrate the principles already indicated, we will consider some specific problems together with suggestive treatment for each.

[Footnote A: Jean Paul Richter, "Der einsige." German writer and philosopher. His rather whimsical and fragmentary book on education, called "Levana," contains some rare scraps of wisdom much used by later writers on educational topics.] [Footnote B: Herbert Spencer, English Philosopher and Scientist. His book on "Education" is sound and practical.] [Footnote C: Freidrich Froebel, German Philosopher and Educator, founder of the Kindergarten system, and inaugurator of the new education. His two great books are "The Education of Man" and "The Mother Play."] [Footnote D: "The Ordeal of Richard Feveril," by George Meredith.] [Footnote E: Tiedemann, German Psychologist.]

[A]

> Jean Paul Richter, "Der einsige." German writer and philosopher. His rather whimsical and fragmentary book on education, called "Levana," contains some rare scraps of wisdom much used by later writers on educational topics.

[B]

> Herbert Spencer, English Philosopher and Scientist. His book on "Education" is sound and practical.

[C]

> Freidrich Froebel, German Philosopher and Educator, founder of the Kindergarten system, and inaugurator of the new education. His two great books are "The Education of Man" and "The Mother Play."

[D]

> "The Ordeal of Richard Feveril," by George Meredith.

[E]

> Tiedemann, German Psychologist.

QUICK TEMPER.

This, as well as irritability and nervousness, very often springs from a wrong physical condition. The digestion may be bad, or the child may be overstimulated. He may not be sleeping enough, or may not get enough outdoor air and exercise. In some cases the fault appears because the child lacks the discipline of young companionship. Even the most exemplary adult cannot make up to the child for the influence of other children. He perceives the difference between himself and these giants about him, and the perception sometimes makes him furious. His struggling individuality finds it difficult to maintain itself under the pressure of so many stronger personalities. He makes, therefore, spasmodic and violent attempts of self-assertion, and these attempts go under the name of fits of temper.

The child who is not ordinarily strong enough to assert himself effectively will work himself up into a passion in order to gain strength, much as men sometimes stimulate their courage by liquor. In fact, passion is a sort of moral intoxication.

Remedy—Solitude and Quiet

But whether the fits of passion are physical or moral, the immediate remedy is the same—his environment must be promptly changed and his audience removed. He needs solitude and quiet. This does not mean shutting him into a closet, but leaving him alone in a quiet room, with plenty of pleasant things about. This gives an opportunity for the disturbed organism to right itself, and for the will to recover its normal tone. Some occupation should be at hand—blocks or other toys, if he is too young to read; a good book or two, such as Miss Alcott's "Little Men" and "Little Women," when he is old enough to read.

If he is destructive in his passion, he must be put in a room where there are very few breakables to tempt him. If he does break anything he must be required to help mend it again. To shout a threat to this effect through the door when the storm of temper is still on, is only to goad him into fresh acts of rebellion. Let him alone while he is in this temporarily insane state, and later, when he is sorry and wants to be good, help him to repair the mischief he has wrought. It is as foolish to argue with or to threaten the child in this state as it would be were he a patient in a lunatic asylum.

It is sometimes impossible to get an older child to go into retreat. Then, since he cannot be carried, and he is not open to remonstrance or commands, go out of the room yourself and leave him alone there. At any cost, loneliness and quiet must be brought to bear upon him.

Such outbursts are exceedingly exhausting, using up in a few minutes as much energy as would suffice for many days of ordinary activity. After the attack the child needs rest, even sleep, and usually seeks it himself. The desire should be encouraged.

Precautions to be Taken

Every reasonable precaution should be taken against the recurrence of the attacks, for every lapse into this excited state makes him more certain the next lapse and weakens the nervous control. This does not mean that you should give up any necessary or right regulations for fear of the child's temper. If the child sees that you do this, he will on occasion deliberately work himself up into a passion in order to get his own way. But while you do not relax any just regulations, you may safely help him to meet them. Give him warning. For instance, do not spring any disagreeable commands upon him. Have his duties as systematized as possible so that he may know what to expect; and do not under any circumstances nag him nor allow other children to tease him.

SULLENNESS.

This fault likewise often has a physical cause, seated very frequently in the liver. See that the child's food is not too heavy. Give him much fruit, and insist upon vigorous exercise out of doors. Or he may perhaps not have enough childish pleasures. For while most children are overstimulated, there still remain some children whose lives are unduly colorless and eventless. A sullen child is below the normal level of responsiveness. He needs to be roused, wakened, lifted out of himself, and made to take an active interest in other persons and in the outside world.

Inheritance and Example

In many cases sullenness is an inherited disposition intensified by example. It is unchildlike and morbid to an unusual degree and very difficult to cure. The mother of a sullen child may well look to her own conduct and examine with a searching eye the peculiarities of her own family and of her husband's. She may then find the cause of the evil, and by removing the child from the bad example and seeing to it that every day contains a number of childish pleasures, she may win him away from a fault that will otherwise cloud his whole life.

LYING.

All lies are not bad, nor all liars immoral. A young child who cannot yet understand the obligations of truthfulness cannot be held morally accountable for his departure from truth. Lying is of three kinds.

(1.) *The imaginative lie.* (2.) *The evasive lie.* (3.) *The politic lie.*

Imaginative "Lying"

(1.) It is rather hard to call the imaginative lie a lie at all. It is so closely related to the creative instinct which makes the poet and novelist and which, common among the peasantry of a nation, is responsible for folk-lore and mythology, that it is rather an intellectual activity misdirected than a moral obliquity. Very imaginative children often do not know the difference between what they imagine and what they actually see. Their minds eye sees as vividly as their bodily eye; and therefore they even believe their own statements. Every attempt at contradiction only brings about a fresh assertion of the impossible, which to the child becomes more and more certain as he hears himself affirming its existence.

Punishment is of no use at all in the attempt to regulate this exuberance. The child's large statements should be smiled at and passed over. In the meantime, he should be encouraged in every possible way to get a firm, grasp of the actual world about him. Manual training, if it can be obtained, is of the greatest advantage, and for a very young child, the performance every day of some little act, which demands accuracy and close attention, is necessary. For the rest, wait; this is one of the faults that disappear with age.

The Lie of Evasion

(2.) The lie of evasion is a form of lying which seldom appears when the relations between child and parents are absolutely friendly and open. However, the child who is very desirous of approval may find it difficult to own up to a fault, even when he is certain that the consequence of his offense will not be at all terrible. This is the more difficult, because the more subtle condition. It is obvious that the child who lies merely to avoid punishment can be cured of that fault by removing from him the fear of punishment. To this end, he should be informed that there will be no punishment whatever for any fault that he freely confesses. For the chief object of punishment being to make him face his own fault and to see it as something ugly and disagreeable, that object is obviously accomplished by a free and open confession, and no further punishment is required.

But when the child in spite of such reassurance still continues to lie, both because he cannot bear to have you think him capable of wrong-doing, and because he is not willing to acknowledge to himself that he is capable of wrong-doing, the situation becomes more complex. All you can do is to urge upon him the superior beauty of frankness; to praise him and love him, especially when he does acknowledge a fault, thus leading him to see that the way to win your approval—that approval which he desires so intensely—is to face his own shortcomings with a steady eye and confess them to you unshrinkingly.

The Politic Lie

(3.) The politic lie is of course the worst form of lying, partly because it is so unchildlike. This is the kind of fault that will grow with age; and grow with such rapidity that the mother must set herself against it with all the force at her command. The child who lies for policy's sake, in order to achieve some end which is most easily achieved by lying, is a child led into wrong-doing by his ardent desire to get something or do something. Discover what this something is, and help him to get it by more legitimate means. If you point out the straight path, and show the goal well in view, at the end of it, he may be persuaded not to take the crooked path.

Inherited Crookedness

But there are occasionally natures that delight in crookedness and that even in early childhood. They would rather go about getting their heart's desire in some crooked, intricate, underhanded way than by the direct route. Such a fault is almost certain to be an inherited one; and here again, a close study of the child's relatives will often help the mother to make a good diagnosis, and even suggest to her the line of treatment.

Extreme Cases

In an extreme case, the family may unite in disbelieving the child who lies, not merely disbelieving him, when he is lying, but disbelieving him all the time, no matter what he says. He must be made to see, and, that without room for any further doubt, that the crooked paths that he loves do not lead to the goal his heart desires, but away from it. His words, not being true to the facts, have lost their value, and no one around him listens to them. He is, as it were, rendered speechless, and his favorite means of getting his own way is thus made utterly valueless. Such a remedy is in truth a terrible one. While it is being administered, the child suffers to the limit of his endurance; and it is only justified in an extreme case, and after the failure of all gentler means.

JEALOUSY.

Justice and Love

Too often this deadly evil is encouraged in infancy, instead of being promptly uprooted as it ought to be. It is very amusing, if one does not consider the consequences, to sec a little child slap and push away the father or the older brother, who attempts to kiss the mother; but this is another fault that grows with years, and a fault so deadly that once firmly rooted it can utterly destroy the beauty and happiness of an otherwise lovely nature. The first step toward overcoming it must be to make the reign of strict justice in the home so obvious as to remove all excuse for the evil. The second step is to encourage the child's love for those very persons of whom he is most likely to be jealous. If he is jealous of the baby, give him special care of the baby. Jealousy indicates a temperament overbalanced emotionally; therefore, put your force upon the upbuilding of the child's intellect. Give him responsibilities, make him think out things for himself. Call upon him to assist in the family conclaves. In every way cultivate his power of judgment. The whole object of the treatment should be to strengthen his intellect and to accustom his emotions to find outlet in wholesome, helpful activity.

One wise mother made it a rule to pet the next to the baby. The baby, she said, was bound to be petted a good deal because of its helplessness and sweetness, therefore she made a conscious effort to pet the next to the youngest, the one who had just been crowded out of the warm nest of mother's lap by the advent of the newcomer. Such a rule would go far to prevent the beginnings of jealousy.

SELFISHNESS.

This is a fault to which strong-willed children are especially liable. The first exercise of will-power after it has passed the stage of taking possession of the child's own organism usually brings him into conflict with those about him. To succeed in getting hold of a thing against the wish of someone else, and to hold on to it when someone else wants it, is to win a victory. The coveted object becomes dear, not so much for its own sake, as because it is a trophy. Such a child knows not the joy of sharing; he knows only the joys of wresting victory against odds. This is indeed an evil that grows with the years. The child who holds onto his apple, his Candy, or toy, fights tooth and nail everyone who wants to take it from him, and resists all coaxing, is liable to become a hard, sordid, grasping man, who stops at no obstacle to accomplish his purpose.

Yet in the beginning, this fault often hides itself and escapes attention. The selfish child may be quiet, clean, and under ordinary circumstances, obedient. He may not even be quarrelsome; and may therefore come under a much less degree of discipline than his obstreperous, impulsive, rebellious little brother. Yet, in reality, his condition calls for much more careful attention than does the condition of the younger brother.

The Only Child

However, the child who has no brother at all, either older or younger, nor any sister, is almost invited by the fact of his isolation to fall into this sin. Only children may be—indeed, often are—precocious, bright, capable, and well-mannered, but they are seldom spontaneously generous. Their own small selves occupy an undue proportion of the family horizon, and therefore of their own.

Kindergarten a Remedy

This is where the Kindergarten has its great value. In the true Kindergarten the children live under a dispensation of loving justice, and selfishness betrays itself instantly there, because it is alien to the whole spirit of the place. Showing itself, it is promptly condemned, and the child stands convicted by the only tribunal whose verdict really moves him—a jury of his peers. Normal children hate selfishness and condemn it, and the selfish child himself, following the strong, childish impulse of imitation, learns to hate his own fault; and so quick is the forgiveness of children that he needs only to begin to repent before the circle of his mates receives him again.

This is one reason why the Kindergarten takes children at such an early age. Aiming, as it does, to lay the foundations for right thinking and feeling, it must begin before wrong foundations are too deeply laid. Its gentle, searching methods straighten the strong will that is growing crooked, and strengthen the enfeebled one.

Intimate Association a Help

But if the selfish child is too old for the Kindergarten, he should belong to a club. Consistent selfishness will not long be tolerated here. The tacit or outspoken rebuke of his mates has many times the force of a domestic rebuke; because thereby he sees himself, at least for a time, as his comrades see him, and never thereafter entirely loses his suspicion that they may be right. Their individual judgment he may defy, but their collective judgment has in it an almost magical power, and convinces him in spite of himself.

Cultivate Affections

Whatever strong affections the selfish boy shows most be carefully cultivated. Love for another is the only sure cure for selfishness. If he loves animals, let him have pets, and give into his hands the whole responsibility for the care of them. It is better to let the poor animals suffer some neglect, than to take away from the boy the responsibility for their condition. They serve him only so far as he can be induced to serve them. The chief rule for the cure of selfishness is, then, to watch every affection, small and large, encourage it, give it room to grow, and see to it that the child does not merely get delight out of it, but that he works for it, that he sacrifices himself for those whom he loves.

LAZINESS.

The Physical Cause

This condition is often normal, especially during adolescence. The developing boy or girl wants to lop and to lounge, to lie sprawled over the floor or the sofa. Quick movement is distasteful to him, and often has an undue effect upon the heart's action. He is normally dreamy, languid, indifferent, and subject to various moods. These things are merely tokens of the tremendous change that is going on within his organism, and which heavily drains his vitality. Certain duties may, of course, be required of him at this stage, but they should be light and steady. He should not be expected to fill up chinks and run errands with joyful alacrity. The six- or eight-year-old may be called upon for these things, and not he harmed, but this is not true of the child between twelve and seventeen. He has absorbing business on hand and should not be too often called away from it.

Laziness and Rapid Growth

Laziness ordinarily accompanies rapid growth of any kind. The unusually large child, even if he has not yet reached the period of adolescence, is likely to be lazy. His nervous energies are deflected to keep up his growth, and his intelligence is often temporarily dulled by the rapidity of his increase in size.

Hurry Not Natural

Moreover, it is not natural for any child to hurry. Hurry is in itself both a result of nervous strain and a cause of it; and grown people whose nerves have been permanently wrenched away from normal quietude and steadiness, often form a habit of hurry which makes them both unfriendly toward children and very bad for children. These young creatures ought to go along through their days rather dreamily and altogether serenely. Every turn of the screw to tighten their nerves makes more certain some form of early nervous breakdown. They ought to have work to do, of course,— enough of it to occupy both mind and body—but it should be quiet, systematic, regular work, much of it performed automatically. Only occasionally should they be required to do things with a conscious effort to attain speed.

Abnormal Laziness

However, there is a degree of laziness difficult of definition which is abnormal; the child fails to perform any work with regularity, and falls behind both at school and at home. This may be the result of (1) *poor assimilation*, (2) *of anaemia*, or it may be (3) *the first symptom of some disease.*

(1.) Poor assimilation may show itself either by (a) thinness and lack of appetite; (b) fat and abnormal appetite; (c) retarded growth; or (d) irregular and poorly made teeth and weak bones.

Anaemia

(2.) Anaemia betrays itself most characteristically by the color of the lips and gums. These, instead of being red, are a pale yellowish pink, and the whole complexion has a sort of waxy pallor. In extreme cases this pallor even becomes greenish. As the disease is accompanied with little pain, and few if any marked symptoms, beyond sleepiness and weakness, it often exists for some time without being suspected by the parents.

(3.) The advent of many other diseases is announced by a languid indifference to surroundings, and a slow response to the customary stimuli. The child's brain seems clouded, and a light form of torpor invades the whole body. The child, who is usually active and interested in things about him, but who loses his activity and becomes dull and irresponsive, should be carefully watched. It may be that he is merely changing his form of growth—*i.e.*, is beginning to grow tall after completion of his period of laying on flesh, or vice versa. Or he may be entering upon the period of adolescence. But if it is neither of these things, a physician should be consulted.

Monotony

A milder degree of laziness may be induced by a too monotonous round of duties. Try changing them. Make them as attractive as possible. For, of course, you do not require him to perform these duties for your sake, whatever you allow him to suppose about it, but chiefly for the sake of their influence on his character. Therefore, if the influence of any work is bad, you will change it, although the new work may not be nearly so much what you prefer to have him do. Whatever the work is, if it is only emptying waste-baskets, don't nag him, merely expect him to do it, and expect it steadily.

Helping

In their earlier years all children love to help mother. They like any piece of real work even better than play. If this love of activity was properly encouraged, if the mother permitted the child to help, even when he succeeded only in hindering, he might well become one those fortunate persons who love to work. This is the real time for preventing laziness. But if this early period has been missed, the next best thing is to take advantage of every spontaneous interest as it arises; to hitch the impulse, as it were, to some task that must be steadily performed. For example, if the child wants to play with tools, help him to make a small water-wheel, or any other interesting contrivance, and keep him at it by various devices until he has brought it to a fair degree of completion Your aim is to stretch his will each time he attempts to do something a little further than it tends to go of itself; to let him work a little past his first impulse, so that he may learn by degrees to work when work is needed, and not only when he feels like it.

UNTIDINESS.

Neatness Not Natural

Essentially a fault of immaturity as this is, we must beware how we measure it by a too severe adult standard. It is not natural for any young creature to take an interest in cleanliness. Even the young animals are cared for in this respect by their parents; the cow licks her calf; the cat, her kittens; and neither calf nor kittens seem to take much interest in the process. The conscious love of cleanliness and order grows with years, and seems to be largely a matter of custom. The child who has always lived in decent surroundings by-and-by finds them necessary to his comfort, and is willing to make a degree of effort to secure them. On the contrary, the street boy who sleeps in his clothes, does not know what it is to desire a well-made bed, and an orderly room.

Remedies

Example

Habit

The obvious method of overcoming this difficulty, then, is not to chide the child for the fault, but to make him so accustomed to pleasant surroundings that he not help but desire them. The whole process of making the child love order is slow but sure. It consists in (1) *Patient waiting on nature*: first, keep the baby himself sweet and clean, washing the young child yourself, two or three times a day, and showing your delight in his sweetness; dressing him so simply that he keeps in respectable order without the necessity of a painful amount of attention. (2) *Example*: He is to be accustomed to orderly surroundings, and though you ordinarily require him to put away some of his things himself, you do also assist this process by putting away a good deal to which you do not call attention. You make your home not only orderly but pretty, and yourself, also, that his love for you may lead him into a love for daintiness. (3) *Habits*: A few set observances may be safely and steadfastly demanded, but these should be *very* few: Such as that he should not come to breakfast without brushing his teeth and combing his hair, or sit down to any meal with unwashed hands. Make them so few that you can be practically certain that they are attended to, for the whole value of the discipline is not in the superior condition of his teeth, but in the habit of mind that is being formed.

IMPUDENCE.

Impudence is largely due to, (1) lack of perception: (2) to bad example and to suggestion; and (3) to a double standard of morality.

Lack of Perception

(1.) In the first place, too much must not be expected of the young savages in the nursery. Remember that the children there are in a state very much more nearly resembling that of savage or half-civilized nation than resembling your own, and that, therefore, while they will undoubtedly take kindly to showy ceremonial, they are not ripe yet for most of the delicate observances. At best, you can only hope to get the crude material of good manners from them. You can hope that they will be in the main kind in intention, and as courteous under provocation as is consistent with their stage of development. If you secure this, you need not trouble yourself unduly over occasional lapses into perfectly innocent and wholesome barbarism.

Good manners are in the main dependent upon quick sympathies, because sympathies develop the perceptions. A child is much less likely to hurt the feelings or shock the sensibilities of a person whom he loves tenderly than of one for whom he cares very little. This is the chief reason why all children are much more likely to be offensive in speech and action before strangers than when alone in the bosom of their families. They are so far from caring what a stranger thinks or feels that they cannot even forecast his displeasure, nor imagine its reaction upon mother or father. The more, then, that the child's sympathies are broadened, the more he is encouraged to take an interest in all people, even strangers, the better mannered will he become.

Bad Example

(2.) Bad example is more common than is usually supposed. Very few parents are consistently courteous toward their children. They permit themselves a sharp tone of voice, and rough and abrupt habits of speech, that would scarcely be tolerated by any adult. Even an otherwise gentle and amiable woman is often disagreeable in her manner toward her children, commanding them to do things in a way well calculated to excite opposition, and rebuking wrong-doing in unmeasured terms. She usually reserves her soft and gentle speeches for her own friends and for her husband's, yet discourtesy cannot begin to harm them as it harms her children.

It is true that the children are often under foot when she is busiest, when, indeed, she is so distracted as to not be able to think about manners, but if she would acknowledge to herself that she ought to be polite, and that when she fails to be, it is because she has yielded to temptation; and if, moreover, she would make this acknowledgment openly to her children and beg their pardon for her sharp words, as she expects them to beg hers, the spirit of courtesy, at any rate, would prevail in her house, and would influence her children. Children are lovingly ready to forgive an acknowledged fault, but keen-eyed beyond belief in detecting a hidden one.

Double Standard

(3.) The most fertile cause of impudence is assumption of a double standard of morality, one for the child and another for the adult. Impudence is, at bottom, the child's perception of this injustice, and his rebellion against it. When to this double standard,—a standard that measures up gossip, for instance, right for the adult and listening to gossip as wrong for the child— when to this is added the assumption of infallibility, it is no wonder that the child fairly rages.

For, if we come to analyze them, what are the speeches which find so objectionable? "Do it yourself, if you are so smart." "Maybe, I am rude, but I'm not any ruder than you are." "I think you are just as mean as mean can be; I wouldn't be so mean!" Is this last speech any worse in reality than "You are a very naughty little girl, and I am ashamed of you," and all sorts of other expressions of candid adverse opinion? Besides these forms of impudence, there is the peculiarly irritating: "Well, you do it yourself; I guess I can if you can."

In all these cases the child is partly it the right. He is stating the feet as he sees it, and violently asserting that you are not privileged to demand more of him than of yourself. The evil comes in through the fact that he is doing it in an ugly spirit. He is not only desirous of stating the truth, but of putting you in the wrong and himself in the right, and if this hurts you, so much the better. All this is because he is angry, and therefor, in impudence, the true evil to be overcome is the evil of anger.

Example

Show him, then, that you are open to correction. Admit the justice of the rebuke as far as you can, and set him an example of careful courtesy and forbearance at the very moment when these traits are most conspicuously lacking in him. If some special point is involved, some question of privilege, quietly, but very firmly, defer the consideration of it until he is master of himself and can discuss the situation with an open mind and in a courteous manner.

CORPORAL PUNISHMENT.

In all these examples, which are merely suggestive, it is impossible to lay down an absolute moral recipe, because circumstances so truly alter cases—in all these no mention is made of corporal punishment. This is because corporal punishment is never necessary, never right, but is always harmful.

Moral Confusion

There are three principal reasons why it should not be resorted to: *First*, because it is indiscriminate. To inflict bodily pain as a consequence of widely various faults, leads to moral confusion. The child who is spanked for lying, spanked for disobedience, and spanked again for tearing his clothes, is likely enough to consider these three things as much the same, as, at any rate, of equal importance, because they all lead to the same result. This is to lay the foundation for a permanent moral confusion, and a man who cannot see the nature of a wrong deed, and its relative importance, is incapable of guiding himself or others. Corporal punishment teaches a child nothing of the reason why what he does is wrong. Wrong must seem to him to be dependent upon the will of another, and its disagreeable consequences to be escapable if only he can evade the will of that other.

Fear versus Love

Second: Corporal punishment is wrong because it inculcates fear of pain as the motive for conduct, instead of love of righteousness. It tends directly to cultivate cowardice, deceitfulness, and anger—three faults worse than almost any fault against which it can be employed. True, some persons grow up both gentle and straightforward in spite of the fact that they have been whipped in their youth, but it is in spite of, and not because of it. In their homes other good qualities must have counteracted the pernicious effect of this mistaken procedure.

Sensibilities Blunted

Third: Corporal punishment may, indeed, achieve immediate results such as seem at the moment to be eminently desirable. The child, if he be young enough, weak enough, and helpless enough, may be made to do almost anything by fear of the rod; and some of the things he may thus be made to do may be exactly the things that he ought to do; and this certainty of result is exactly what prompts many otherwise just and thoughtful persons to the use of corporal punishment. But these good results are obtained at the expense of the future. The effect of each spanking is a little less than the effect of the preceding one. The child's sensibilities blunt. As in the case of a man with the drug habit, it requires a larger and larger dose to produce the required effect. That is, if he is a strong child capable of enduring and resisting much. If, on the contrary, he is a weak child, whose slow budding will come only timidly into existence, one or two whippings followed by threats, may suffice to keep him in a permanently cowed condition, incapable of initiative, incapable of spontaneity.

The method of discipline here indicated, while it is more searching than any corporal punishment, does not have any of its disadvantages. It is more searching, because it never blunts the child's sensibilities, but rather tends to refine them, and to make them more responsive.

Educative Discipline

Permanent Results

The child thus trained should become more susceptible, day by day, to gentle and elevating influences. This discipline is educative, explaining to the child why what he does is wrong, showing him the painful effects as inherent in the deed itself. He cannot, therefore, conceive of himself as being ever set free from the obligation to do right; for that obligation within his experience does not rest upon his mother's will or ability to inflict punishment, but upon the very nature of the universe of which he is a part. The effects of such discipline are therefore permanent. That which happens to the child in the nursery, also happens to him in the great world when he reaches manhood. His nursery training interprets and orders the world for him. He comes, therefore, into the world not desiring to experiment with evil, but clear-eyed to detect it, and strong-armed to overcome it.

We are now ready to consider our subject in some of its larger aspects.

TEST QUESTIONS

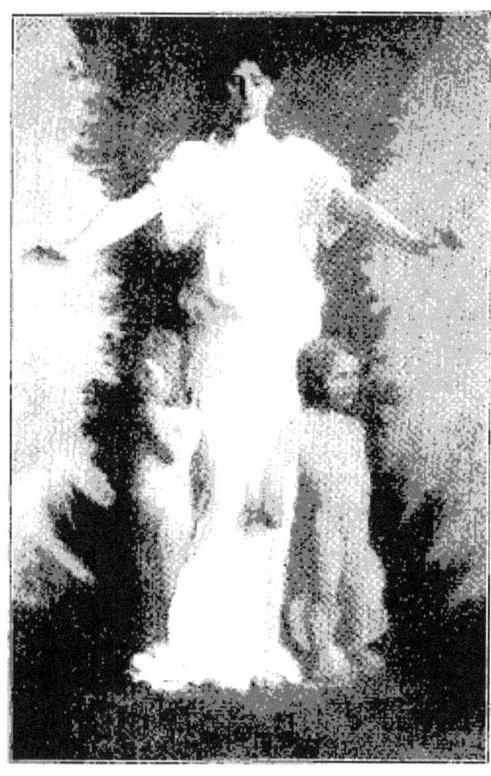

"CARITAS"
From a Painting in the Boston Public Library, by Abbot H. Thayer

The following questions constitute the "written recitation" which the regular members of the A.S.H.E. answer in writing and send in for the correction and comment of the instructor. They are intended to emphasize and fix in the memory the most important points in the lesson.

STUDY OF CHILD LIFE.

PART I.

Read Carefully. In answering these questions you are earnestly requested *not* to answer according to the text-book where opinions are asked for, but to answer according to conviction. In all cases credit will be given for thought and original observation. Place your name and full address at the head of the paper; use your own words so that your instructor may be sure that you understand the subject.

1. How does Fiske account for the prolonged helplessness of the human infant? To what practical conclusions does this lead?

2. Name the four essentials for proper bodily growth.

3. How does the child's world differ from that of the adult?

4. In training a child morally, how do you know which faults are the most important and should have, therefore, the chief attention?

5. In training the will, what end must be held steadily in view?

6. What are the advantages or disadvantages of a broken will?

7. Is obedience important? Obedience to what? How do you train for prompt obedience in emergencies?

8. What is the object of punishment? Does corporal punishment accomplish this object?

9. What kind of punishment is most effective?

10. Have any faults a physical origin? If so, name some of them and explain.

11. What are the two great teachers according to Tiederman?

12. What can you say of the fault of untidiness?

13. What are the dangers of precocity?

14. What do you consider were the errors your own parents made in training their children?

15. Are there any questions which you would like to ask in regard to the subjects taken up in this lesson?

NOTE.—After completing the test, sign your full name.

STUDY OF CHILD LIFE

PART II.

CHARACTER BUILDING

Froebel's Philosophy

Although we have taken up the question of punishment and the manner of dealing with various childish iniquities before the question of character-building, it has only been done in order to clear the mind of some current misconceptions. In the statements of Froebel's simple and positive philosophy of child culture, misconception on the part of the reader must be guarded against, and these misconceptions generally arise from a feeling that, beautiful as his optimistic philosophy may be, there are some children too bad to profit by it—or at least that there are occasions when it will not work out in practice. In the preceding section we have endeavored to show in detail how this method applies to a representative list of faults and shortcomings, and having thus, we hope, proved that the method is applicable to a wide range of cases—indeed to all possible cases—we will proceed to recount the fundamental principles which Froebel, and before him Pestalozzi, [A] enunciated; which times who adhere to the new education are to-day working out into the detail of school-room practice.

Object of Moral Training.

As previously stated, the object of the moral training of the child is the inculcation of the love of righteousness. Froebel is not concerned with laying down a mass of observances which the child must follow, and which the parents must insist upon. He thinks rather that the child's nature once turned into the right direction and surrounded by right influences will grow straight without constant yankings and twistings. The child who loves to do right is safe. He may make mistakes as to what the right is, but he will learn by these mistakes, and will never go far astray.

The Reason Why

However, it is well to save him as far as possible from the pain of these mistakes. We need to preserve in him what has already been implanted there; the love of understanding the reasons for conduct. When the child asks "Why?" therefore, he should seldom be told "Because mother says so."

This is to deny a rightful activity of his young mind; to give him a monotonous and insufficient reason, temporary in its nature, instead of a lasting reason which will remain with him through life. Dante says all those who have lost what he calls "the good of the intellect" are in the Inferno. And when you refuse to give your child satisfactory reasons for the conduct you require of him, you refuse to cultivate in him that very good of the intellect which is necessary for his salvation.

Advantage of Positive Commands

As soon, however, as your commands become positive instead of negative, the difficulty of meeting the situation begins to disappear. It is usually much easier to tell the child why he should do a thing than why he should not do its opposite. For example, it is much easier to make him see that he ought to be a helpful member of the family than to make him understand why he should stop making a loud noise, or refrain from waking up the baby. There is something in the child which in calm moments recognizes that love demands some sacrifice. To this something you must appeal and these calm moments, for the most part, you must choose for making the appeal. The effort is to prevent the appearance of evil by the active presence of good. The child who is busy trying to be good has little time to be naughty.

Original Goodness

Froebel's most characteristic utterance is perhaps this: "A suppressed or perverted good quality—a good tendency, only repressed, misunderstood, or misguided—lies originally at the bottom of every shortcoming in man. Hence the only and infallible remedy for counteracting any shortcoming and even wickedness is to find the originally good source, the originally good side of the human being that has been repressed, disturbed, or misled into the shortcoming, and then to foster, build up, and properly guide this good side. Thus the shortcoming will at last disappear, although it may involve a hard struggle against habit, but not against original depravity in man, and this is accomplished so much the more rapidly and surely because man himself tends to abandon his shortcomings, for man prefers right to wrong." The natural deduction from this is that we should say "do" rather than "don't"; open up the natural way for rightful activity instead of uttering loud warning cries at the entrance to every wrong path.

Kindergarten Methods

It is for this reason that the kindergarten tries by every means to make right doing delightful. This is one of the reasons for its songs, dances, plays, its bright colors, birds, and flowers. And in this respect it may well be imitated in every home. No one loves that which is disagreeable, ugly, and forbidding; yet many little children are expected to love right doing which is seldom attractively presented to them.

The results of such treatment are apparent in the grown people of to-day. Most persons have an underlying conviction that sinners, or at any rate unconscientious persons, have a much easier and pleasanter time of it than those who try to do right. To the imagination of the majority of adults sin is dressed in glittering colors and virtue in gray, somber garments. There are few who do not take credit for right doing as if they had chosen a hard and disagreeable part instead of the more alluring ways of wrong. This is because they have been mis-taught in childhood and have come to think of wrongdoing as pleasant and virtue as hard, whereas the real truth is exactly the opposite. It is wrongdoing that brings unpleasant consequences and virtue that brings happiness.

Right Doing Made Easy

There are those who object that by the kindergarten method right doing is made too easy. The children do not have to put forth enough effort, they say; they are not called upon to endure sufficient pain; they do not have the discipline which causes them to choose right no matter how painful right may be for the moment. Whether this dictum is ever true or not, it certainly is not true in early childhood. The love of righteousness needs to be firmly rooted in the character before it is strained and pulled upon. We do not start seedlings in the rocky soil or plant out saplings in time of frost. If tests and trials of virtue must come, let them come in later life when the love of virtue is so firmly established that it may be trusted to find a way to its own satisfaction through whatever difficulties may oppose.

Neighbors' Opinions

In the very beginning of any effort to live up to Froebel's requirements it is evident that children must not be measured by the way they appear to the neighbors. This is to reaffirm the power of that rigid tradition which has warped so many young lives. She who is trying to fix her child's heart upon true and holy things may well disregard her neighbor's comments on the child's manners or clothes or even upon momentary ebullitions of temper. She is working below the surface of things, is setting eternal forces to work, and she cannot afford to interrupt this work for the sake of shining the child up with any premature outside polish. If she is to have any peace of mind or to allow any to the child, if she is to live in any way a simple and serene life, she must establish a few fundamental principles by which she judges her child's conduct and regulates her own, and stand by these principles through thick and thin.

The Family Republic

Perhaps the most fundamental principle is that enunciated by Fichte. "Each man," he says, "is a free being in a world of other free beings." Therefore his freedom is limited only by the freedom of the other free beings. That is, they must "divide the world amongst them." Stated in the form of a command he says again, "Restrict your freedom through the freedom of all other persons with whom you come in contact." This is a rule that even a three-year-old child can be made to understand, and it is astonishing with what readiness he will admit its justice. He call do anything he wants to, you explain to him, except bother other people. And, of course, the corollary follows that every one else can do whatever he pleases except to bother the child.

Rights of Others

This clear and simple doctrine can be driven home with amazing force, if you strictly respect the child's right as you require him to respect yours. You should neither allow any encroachments upon your own proper privileges, except so far as you explain that this is only a loving permission on your part, and not to be assumed as a precedent or to be demanded as a right; nor should you yourself encroach upon his privileges.

If you do not expect him to interrupt you, you must not interrupt him. If you expect him to let you alone when you are busy, you must let hint alone when he is busy, that is, when he is hard at work playing. If you must call him away from his playing, give him warning, so that he may have time to put his small affairs in order before obeying your command. The more carefully you do this the more willing will be his response on the infrequent occasions when you must demand immediate attention. In some such fashion you teach the child to respect the rights of others by scrupulously respecting those rights to which he is most alive, namely, his own. The next step is to require him with you to think out the rights of others, and both of you together should shape your conduct so as to leave these rights unfringed.

The Child's Share in Ruling

As soon as the young child's will has fully taken possession of his own organism he will inevitably try to rule yours. The establishment of the law of which I have just spoken will go far toward regulating this new-born desire. But still he must be allowed in some degree to rule others, because power to rule others is likely to be at some time during his life of great importance to him. To thwart him absolutely in this respect, never yielding yourself to his imperious demands, is alike impossible and undesirable. His will must not be shut up to himself and to the things that he can make himself do. In various ways, with due consideration for other people's feelings, with courtesy, with modesty, he may well be encouraged to do his share of ruling. And while, of course, he will not begin his ruling in such restrained and thoughtful fashion as is implied by these limitations, yet he must be suffered to begin; and the rule for the respect of the rights of others should be suffered gradually to work out these modifications.

A safe distinction may be made as follows: Permit him, since he is so helpless, to rule and persuade others to satisfy his legitimate desires, such as the desire for food, sleep, affection, and knowledge; but when be demands indulgencies, reserve your own liberty of choice, so as to clearly demonstrate to him that you are exercising choice, and in doing so, are well within your own rights.

Low Voice Commands

There is one simple outward observation which greatly assists us the inculcation of these fundamental truths—that is the habit of using a low voice in speaking, especially when issuing a command or administering a rebuke. A loud, insistent voice practically insures rebellion. This is because the low voice means that you have command of yourself, the loud voice that you have lost it. The child submits to a controlled will, but not to one as uncontrolled as his own. In both cases he follows your example. If you are self-controlled, he tends to become so; if you are excited and angry, he also becomes so, or if he is already so, his excitement and anger increases.

While most mothers rely altogether too much upon speech as a means of explaining life to the child, yet it must be admitted that speech has a great function to perform in this regard. Nevertheless it is well to bear in mind that it is not true that a child will always do what you tell him to do, no matter how plain you may tell him, nor how perfectly you may explain your reasons.

Limitations of Words

In the first place, speech means less to children than to grown persons. Each word has a smaller content of experience. They cannot get the full force of the most clear and eloquent statement. Therefore all speech must be reinforced by example, and by as many forms of concrete illustrations as can be commanded. Each necessary truth should enter the child's mind by several channels; hearing, eye-sight, motor activity should all be called upon. Many truths may be dramatized. This, where the mother is clever enough to employ it, is the surest method of appeal. But in any case, speech alone must not be relied upon, nor the child considered a hopeless case who does not respond to it.

Denunciatory speech especially needs wise regulation. As Richter says, "What is to be followed as a rule of prudence, yea, of justice, toward grown-up people, should be much more observed toward children, namely, that one should never judgingly declare, for instance, 'You are a liar,' or even, 'You are a bad boy,' instead of saying, 'You have told an untruth,' or 'You have done wrong.' For since the power to command yourself implies at the same time the power of obeying, man feels a minute after his fault as free as Socrates, and the branding mark of his *nature*, not his *deed*, must seem to him blameworthy of punishment.

"To this must be added that every individual's wrong actions, owing to his inalienable sense of a moral aim and hope, seem to him only short, usurped interregnums of the devil, or comets in the uniform solar system. The child, consequently, under such a moral annihilation, feels the wrong-doing of others more than his own; and this all the more because, in him, want of reflection and the general warmth of his feelings, represent the injustice of others in a more ugly light than his own."

Example versus Precept

If any one desires to prove the superior force of example over precept, let him try teaching a baby to say "Thank you" or "Please," merely by being scrupulously careful to say these things to the baby on all fit occasions. No one has taken the statistics of the number of times every small child is exhorted to perfect himself in this particular observance; but it is safe to say that in the United States alone these injunctions are spoken something like a million times a day and all quite unnecessarily. The child will say "Please" and "Thank you" without being told to do so, if he merely has his attention called to the fact that the people around him all use these phrases.

Politeness to Children

The truth is, too many parents forget to speak these agreeable words whenever they ask favors of their own children; so the force of their example is marred. What you do to the child himself, remember, always outweighs anything you do to others before him. This is the reason why it is necessary that you should acknowledge your own shortcomings to the child, if you expect him to acknowledge his to you. It is also necessary sometimes to point out clearly the kind and considerate things that you are in the habit of doing to others, lest the untrained mind of the young child may fail to see and so miss the force of your example.

But in thus revealing your own good deeds to the child, remember the motive, and reveal them only (a) when he cannot perceive them of himself, (b) when he needs to perceive them in order that his own conduct may be influenced by them, and (c) at the time when he is most likely to appreciate them. This latter requirement precludes you from announcing your own righteousness when he is naughty, and compels you, of course, to go directly against your native impulse, which is to mention your deeds of sacrifice and kindness only when you are angry and mean to reproach him with them. When you tell him how devoted you have been at some moment when you are both thoroughly angry, he is in danger of either denying or hating your devotion; but when you refer to it tenderly, and, as your heart will then prompt you, modestly, at some loving moment, he will give it recognition, and be moved to love goodness more devotedly because you embody it.

Law-Making Habit

Another important rule is this: Do not make too many rules. Some women are like legislatures in perpetual session. The child who is confused and tantalized by the constant succession of new laws learns presently to disregard them, and to regulate his life according to certain deductions of his own—sometimes surprisingly wise and politic deductions. The way to re yourself of this law-making habit is to stop thinking of every little misdeed as the beginning of a great wrong. It is very likely an accident and a combination of circumstances such as may not happen again. To treat misdemeanors which are not habitual nor characteristic as evanescent is the best way to make them evanescent. They should not be allowed to enter too deeply into your consciousness or into that of your child.

Live with Your Children

In order to be able to discriminate between accidental wrong-doing, and that which is the first symptom of wrong-thinking, you must be in close touch with your children. This brings us to Froebel's great motto, "Come, let us live with our children!" This means that you are not merely to talk with your child, to hear from his lips what he is doing, but to live so closely with him, that in most cases you know what he is doing without any need of his telling you. When, however, he does tell you something which happened in the school play-ground or otherwise out of the range of your knowledge, be careful not to moralize over it. Make yourself as agreeable a secret-keeper as his best friend of his own age; let your moralizing be so rare that it is effective for that very reason. If the occasion needs moral reflection at all—and that seldom happens—the wise way is to lead the child to do his own reflecting; to arrive at his own conclusions, and if you must lead him, by all means do so as invisibly as possible. For the most part it is safe to take the confessions lightly, and well to keep your own mind young by looking at things from the boy's point of view.

The Subject of Sex

If, however, there is to be perfect confidence between you, the one subject which is usually kept out of speech between mothers and children must be no forbidden subject between them; you must not refuse to answer questions about the mystery of sex. If you are not the fit person to teach your child these important facts, who is? Certainly not the school-mates and servants from whom he is likely to learn them if you refuse to furnish the information. Usually it is sufficient simply to answer the child's honest questions honestly; but any mother who finds herself unable to cope with this simple matter in this simple spirit, will find help in Margaret Morley's "Song of Life," in the Wood-Allen Publications, and the books of the Rev. Sylvanus Stall.[B]

In respect to these matters more than in respect to others, but also in respect to all matters, children often do not know that they are doing wrong, even when it it very difficult for parents to believe that they do not intend wrong-doing. As we have seen from our analysis of truthfulness, the child may very often lie without a qualm of conscience, and he may still more readily break the unwritten rules of courtesy, asking abrupt and even cruel questions of strangers, and haul the family skeleton out of its closet at critical moments. Such things cannot be wholly guarded against, even by the exercise of the utmost wisdom, but the habit of reasoning things out for himself is the greatest help a child can have.

Righteousness

The formation of the bent of the child's nature as a whole is a matter of unconscious education, but as he grows in the power to reason, conscious education must direct his mental activity. It is not enough for him, as it is not enough for any grown person, to do the best that he knows; he must learn to know the best. The word righteousness itself means right-wiseness, i.e., right knowingness.

To quote Froebel again, "In order, therefore, to impart true, genuine firmness to the natural will-activity of the boy, all the activities of the boy, his entire will should proceed from and have reference to the development, cultivation, and representation of the internal. Instruction in example and in words, which later on become precept and example, furnishes the means for this. Neither example alone, nor words will do; not example alone, for it is particular and special, and the word is needed to give the particular individual example universal applicability; not words alone, for example is needed to interpret and explain the word, which is general, spiritual, and of many meanings.

"But instruction and example alone and in themselves are not sufficient; they must meet a good pure heart and this is the outcome of proper educational influences in childhood."

Moral Precocity

Lest these directions should seem to demand an almost superhuman degree of control and wisdom on the part of the mother, remember that moral precocity is as much to be guarded against a mental precocity. Remember that you are neither required to be a perfect mother nor to rear a perfect child. As Spencer remarks, a perfect child in this imperfect world would be sadly out of joint with the times, would indeed be a martyr. If your basic principles are right and if your child has before him the daily and hourly spectacle of a mother who is trying to conform herself to high standards, he will grow as fast as it is safe for him to grow. Spencer says: "Our higher moral faculties like our higher intellectual ones, are comparatively complex. As a consequence they are both comparatively late in their evolution, and with the one as with the other, a very early activity produced by stimulation will be at the expense of the future character. Hence the not uncommon fact that those who during childhood were instanced as models of juvenile goodness, by and by undergo some disastrous and seemingly inexplicable change, and end by being not above but below par; while relatively exemplary men are often the issue of a childhood not so promising.

"Be content, therefore, with moderate measures and moderate results, constantly bearing in mind the fact that the higher morality, like the higher intelligence, must be reached by a slow growth; and you will then have more patience with those imperfections of nature which your child hourly displays. You will be less prone to constant scolding, and threatening, and forbidding, by which many parents induce a chronic irritation, in a foolish hope that they will thus make their children what they should be."

Rules in Character Building

In conclusion, the rules that may be safely followed in character-building may be summed up thus:

(1) Recognize that the object of your training is to help the child to love righteousness. Command little and then use positive commands rather than prohibitions. Use "do" rather than "don't."

(2) Make right-doing delightful.

(3) Establish Fichte's doctrine of right, see page 64.

(4) Teach by example rather than precept. Therefore respect the child's rights as you wish him to respect yours.

(5) Use a low voice, especially in commanding or rebuking.

(6) In chiding, remember Richter's rule and rebuke the sin and not the sinner.

(7) Confess your own misdeeds, by this means and others securing the confidence of your children.

Finally, remember that this is an imperfect world, you are an imperfect mother, and the best results you can hope for are likely to be imperfect. But the results may be so founded upon eternal principles as to tend continually to give place to better and better results.

[A]

>Pestalozzi, Educator, Philosopher, and Reformer. Author of "How Gertrude Teaches Her Children."

[B]

>"What a Young Girl Ought to Know" and "What a Young Woman Ought to Know" by Dr. Mary Wood Allen. "What a Young Boy Ought to Know," "What a Young Man Ought to Know," by Rev. Sylvanus Stall.

PLAY

Although Froebel is best known as the educator who first took advantage of play as a means of education, he was not, in reality, the first to recognize the high value of this spontaneous activity. He was indeed the first to put this recognition into practice and to use the force generated during play to help the child to a higher state of knowledge.

But before him Plato said that the plays of children have the mightiest influence on the maintenance or the non-maintenance of laws; that during the first three years the child should be made "cheerful" and "kind" by having sorrow and fear and pain kept away from him and by soothing him with music and rhythmic movements.

Aristotle

Aristotle held that children until they were five years old "should be taught nothing, not even necessary labor, lest it hinder growth, but should be accustomed to use much motion as to avoid a indolent habit of body, and this," he added, "can he acquired by various means, among others by play, which ought to be neither illiberal, nor laborious, or lazy."

Luther

Luther rebukes those who despise the plays of children and says that Solomon did not prohibit scholars from play at the proper time. Fenelon, Locke, Schiller, and Richter all admit the deep significance of this universal instinct of youth.

Preyer, speaking not as a philosopher or educator, but as a scientist, mentions "the new kinds of pleasurable sensations with some admixture of intellectual elements," which are gained when the child gradually begins to play. Much that is called play he considers true experimenting, especially when the child is seen to be studying the changes produced by his own activity, as when he tears paper into small bits, shakes a bunch of keys, opens and shuts a box, plays with sand, and empties bottles, and throws stones into the water. "The zeal with which these seemingly aimless movements are executed is remarkable. The sense of gratification must be very great, and is principally due to the feeling of his own power, and of being the cause of the various changes."

Educational Value of Play

All these authorities are quoted here in order to show that the practical recognition of play which obtains among the advanced educators to-day is not a piece of sentimentalism, as stern critics sometimes declare, but the united opinion of some of the wisest minds of this and former ages. As Froebel says, "Play and speech constitute the element in which the child lives. At this stage (the first three years of childhood) he imparts to everything the virtues of sight, feeling, and speech. He feels the unity between himself and the whole external world." And Froebel conceives it to be of the profoundest importance that this sense of unity should not be disturbed. He finds that play is the most spiritual activity of man at this age, "and at the same time typical of human life as a whole—of the inner, hidden, natural life of man and all things; it gives, therefore, joy, freedom, contentment, inner and outer rest, peace with the world: it holds the sources of all that is good. The child that plays thoroughly until physical fatigue forbids will surely be a thorough, determined man, capable of self-sacrifice for the promotion and welfare of himself and others."

But all play does not deserve this high praise. It fits only the play under right conditions. Fortunately these are such that every mother can command them. There are three essentials: (1) Freedom, (2) Sympathy, (3) Right materials.

Freedom

(1) Freedom is the first essential, and here the child of poverty often has the advantage of the child of wealth. There are few things in the poverty-stricken home too good for him to play with; in its narrow quarters, he becomes, perforce, a part of all domestic activity. He learns the uses of household utensils, and his play merges by imperceptible degrees into true, healthful work.

In the home of wealth, however, there is no such freedom, no such richness of opportunity. The child of wealth has plenty of toys, but few real things to play with. He is shut out of the common activity of the family, and shut in to the imitation activity of his nursery. He never gets his small hands on realities, but in his elegant clothes is confined to the narrow conventional round that is falsely supposed to be good for him.

Froebel insists upon the importance of the child's dress being loose, serviceable, and inconspicuous, so that he may play as much as possible without consciousness of the restrictions of dress. The playing child should also have, as we have noticed in the first section, the freedom of the outside world. This does not mean merely that he should go out in his baby-buggy, or take a ride in the park, but that he should be able to play out-of-doors, to creep on the ground, to be a little open-air savage, and play with nature as he finds it.

Sympathy

(2) Sympathy is much more likely to rise spontaneously in the mother's breast for the child's troubles than for the child's joys. She will stop to take him up and pet him when he is hurt, no matter how busy she is, but she too often considers it waste of time to enter into his plays with him; yet he needs sympathy in joy as much as in sorrow. Her presence, her interest in what he is doing, doubles his delight in it and doubles its value to him. Moreover, it offers her opportunity for that touch and direction now and then, which may transform a rambling play, without much sequence or meaning, into a consciously useful performance, a dramatization, perhaps, of some of the child's observations, or an investigation into the nature of things.

(3) Right Material. Even given freedom and sympathy, the child needs something more in order to play well: he needs the right materials. The best materials are those that are common to him and to the rest of the world, far better than expensive toys that mark him apart from the world of less fortunate children. Such toys are not in any way desirable, and they may even be harmful. What he needs are various simple arrangements of the four elements—earth, air, fire and water.

Mud-pies

(1) *Earth*. The child has a noted affinity for it, and he is specially happy when he has plenty of it on hands, face, and clothes. The love of mud-pies is universal; children of all nationalities and of all degrees of civilization delight in it. No activity could be more wholesome.

Sand

Next to mud comes sand. It is cleaner in appearance and can be brought into the house. A tray of moistened sand, set upon a low table, should be in every nursery, and the sand pile in every yard.

Clay

Clay is more difficult to manage indoors, because it gets dry and sifts all about the house, but if a corner of the cellar, where there is a good light, can be given up for a strong table and a jar of clay mixed with some water, it will be found a great resource for rainy days. If modeling aprons of strong material, buttoned with one button at the neck, be hung near the jar of clay, the children may work in this material without spoiling their clothes. Clay-modeling is an excellent form of manual training, developing without forcing the delicate muscles of the fingers and wrists, and giving wide opportunity for the exercise of the imagination.

Digging

Earth may be played with in still another way. Children should dig in it; for all pass through the digging stage and this should be given free swing. It develops their muscles and keeps them busy at helpful and constructive work. They may dig a well, make a cave, or a pond, or burrow underground and make tunnels like a mole. Give them spades and a piece of ground they can do with as they like, dress them in overalls, and it will be long before you are asked to think of another amusement for them.

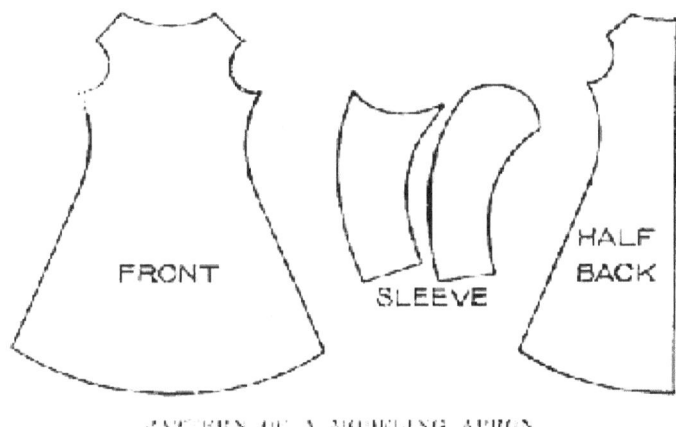

PATTERN OF A MODELING APRON.

Gardens

In still another way the earth may be utilized, for children may make gardens of it. Indeed, there are those who say that no child's education is complete until he has had a garden of his own and grown in it all sorts of seeds from pansies to potatoes. But a garden is too much for a young child to care for all alone. He needs the help, advice, and companionship of some older person. You must be careful, however, to give help only when it is really desired; and careful also not to let him feel that the garden is a task to which he is driven daily, but a joy that draws him.

Kites Windmills Soap-bubbles

(2) *The Air*. The next important plaything is the air. The kite and the balloon are only two instruments to help the child play with it. Little windmills made of colored paper and stuck by means of a pin at the end of a whittled stick, make satisfactory toys. One of their great advantages is that even a very young child can make them for himself. Blowing soap-bubbles is another means of playing with air. By giving the children woolen mittens the bubbles may be caught and tossed about as well as blown.

(3) *Water*. Perhaps the very first thing he learns to play with is water. Almost before he knows the use of his hands and legs he plays with water in his bath, and sucks his sponge with joy, thus feeling the water with his chief organs of touch, his mouth and tongue. A few months later he will be glad to pour water out of a tin cup. Even when he is two or three years old, be may be amused by the hour, by dressing him in a woolen gown, with his sleeves rolled high, and setting him down before a big bowl or his own bath-tub half full of warm water. To this may be added a sponge, a tin cup, a few bits of wood, and some paper. They should not be given all at once, but one at a time, the child allowed to exhaust the possibilities of each before another is added. Still later he may be given the bits of soap left after a cake of soap is used up. Give him also a few empty bottles or bowls and let him put them away with a solid mass of soap-suds in them and see what will happen. When he is older—past the period of putting everything in his mouth—he may be given a few bits of bright ribbons, petals of artificial flowers, or any bright colored bits of cloth which can color the water.

Children love to sprinkle the grass with the hose or to water the flowers with the sprinkling can. They enjoy also the metal fishes, ducks, and boats which may be drawn about in the water by means of a magnet. Presently they reach the stage when they must have toy-boats, and next they long to go into real boats and go rowing and sailing. They want to fish, wade, swim, and skate.

Dangerous Pastimes

Some of those pastimes are dangerous, but they are sure to be indulged in at some time or other, with or without permission. There never grew a child to sturdy manhood who was successfully kept away from water. The wise mother, then, will not forbid this play, but will do her best to regulate it, to make it safe. She will think out plans for permitting children to go swimming in a safe place with some older person. She will let them go wading, and at holiday time will take them boat-riding. If she permits as much activity in these respects as possible, her refusal when it does come will be respected; and the child will not, unless perhaps in the first bitterness of disappointment, think her unfriendly and fussy. Above all, he is not likely to try to deceive her, to run off and take a swim on the sly, and thus fall into true danger.

Precaution with Fire

(4) *Fire* is another inevitable plaything. Miss Shinn reports that the first act of her little niece that showed the dawn of voluntary control of the muscles was the clinging of her eyes to the flame of a candle, at the end of the second week. The sense of light and the pleasure derived from it is of the chief incentives to a baby's intellectual development. But since fire is dangerous the child must be taught this fact as quickly and painlessly as possible. He will probably have to be burned once before he really understands it, but by watching you can make this pain very small and slight, barely sufficient to give the child a wholesome fear of playing with unguarded fire. For instance, show that the lamp globe is hot. It is not hot enough to injure him, but quite hot enough to be unpleasant to his sensitive nerves. Put your own hand on the lamp and draw it away with a sharp cry, saying warningly, "Hot, hot!" Do not put his hand on the lamp, but let him put it there himself and then be very sympathetic over the result. Usually one such lesson is sufficient. Only do not permit yourself to call everything hot which you do not want him to touch. He will soon discover that you are untruthful and will never again trust you so fully.

Bonfires

Under *proper regulations*, however, fire may be played with safely. Bonfires with some older person in attendance are safe enough and prevent unlawful bonfires in dangerous places. The rule should be that none of the children may play with fire except with permission; and then that permission should be granted as often as possible that the children may be encouraged to ask for it. A stick smouldering at one end and waved about in circles and ellipses is not dangerous when elders are by, but it is dangerous if played with on the sly. Playing with fire on the sly is the most dangerous thing a child can do, and the only way to prevent it is to permit him to play with fire in the open. A beautiful game can be made from number of Christmas tree candles of various colors and a bowl of water. The candles are lighted and the wax dropped into the water, making little colored circles which float about. These can be linked together such a fashion as to form patterns which may be lifted out on sheets of paper.

Magic Lantern

The magic lantern is an innocent and comparatively cheap means of playing with light. If it is well taken care of and fresh slides added from time to time it can be made a source of pleasure for years. Jack-o'-lanterns are great fun, and when pumpkins are not available, oranges may be used instead.

Rhythmic Movements

Besides these elemental playthings the child gets much valuable pleasure out of the rhythmic use of his own muscles. All such plays Plato thought should be regulated by music, and with this Froebel agreed, but in the Household this is often impossible. The children must indulge in many movements when there is no one about who has leisure to make music for them. Still, when they come to the quarrelsome age, a few minutes' rhythmic play to the sound of music will be found to harmonize the whole group wonderfully. For this purpose the ordinary hippity-hop, fast or slow according to the music, is sufficient. It is as if the regulation of the body to the laws of harmony reacted upon minds and nerves. Such an exercise is particularly valuable just before bed-time. The children go to sleep then with their minds under the influence of harmony and wake in the morning inclined to be peaceful and happy.

Songs

A book of Kindergarten songs, such as Mrs. Gaynor's "Songs of the Child World" and Eleanor Smith's "Songs for the Children," ought to be in every household, and the mother ought to familiarize herself with a dozen or so of these perfectly simple melodies. Of course the children must learn them with her. When once this has been done she has a valuable means of amusing them and bringing them within her control at any time. She may hum one of the songs or play it. The children must guess what it is and then act out their guess in pantomime, so that she can see what they mean. Perhaps it is a windmill song; their arms fly around and around in time to the music, now fast, now slow. Perhaps it is a Spring song; the children are birds building their nests. Other songs turn them into shoemakers, galloping horses, or soldiers.

Dramatic Plays

Dramatic plays, whether simple, like this, or elaborate, are, as Goethe shows in *Wilhelm Meister,* of the greatest possible educational advantage. In them the child expresses his ideas of the world about him and becomes master of his own ideas. He acts out whatever he has heard or seen. He acts out also whatever he is puzzling about, and by making the terms of his problem clear to his consciousness usually solves it.

Dancing

As for dancing, Richter exclaims: "I know not whether I should most deprecate children's balls or most praise children's dances. For the harmony connected with it (dancing) imparts to the affections and the mind that material order which reveals the highest, and regulates the beat of the pulse, the step, and even the thought. Music is the meter of this poetic movement, and is an invisible dance, as dancing is a silent music. Finally, this also ranks among the advantages of his eye and heel pleasure; that children with children, by no harder canon than the musical, light as sound, may be joined in a rosebud feast without thorns or strife." The dances may be of the simplest kind, such as "Ring Around a Rosy," "Here We Go, To and Fro," "Old Dan Tucker" and the "Virginia Reel." The old-fashioned singing plays, such as "London Bridge," "Where Oats, Peas, Beans, and Barley Grow," and "Pop Goes the Weasel" have their place and value. Several collections of them have been made and published, but usually quite enough material may be found for these plays in the memories of the people of any neighborhood.

Toys

All these plays, it will be noticed, call for very simple and inexpensive apparatus, in most cases for no apparatus at all. Nevertheless there is a place for toys. All children ought to have a few, both because of the innocent pleasure they afford and because they need to have certain possessions which are inalienably their own. A simple and inexpensive list of suitable toys adapted to various ages is given at the end of this section. Most of them are exactly the toys that parents usually buy. But it will be noticed that none of them are very elaborate or expensive, and that the patrol wagon is not among them. This is because the patrol wagon directly leads to plays that are not only uneducational but positively harmful in their tendencies. The children of a whole neighborhood were once led into the habit of committing various imitation crimes for the sake of being arrested and carried off in miniature patrol wagon. It any such expensive and elaborate toys are bought, it may well be the plain express wagon or the hook and ladder and fire engine. The first of these leads to plays of industry, the second to those of heroism.

```
LIST OF TOYS SUITABLE FOR VARIOUS AGES.

Ball, rubber ring, soft animals and rag dolls ......... Before 1 year
Blocks and Bells ............................................. 1 year
Small chair and table ....................................1 1/2 years
Noah's Ark .................................................. 2 years
Picture books ............................................... 2 years
Materials and instruments ............................. 2 to 3 years
Carts, stick-horses, and reins ..................... 2 1/2 to 3 years
Boats, ships, engines, tin or wooden animals, dolls,
dishes, broom, spade, sand-pile, bucket, etc ............... 3 years
Hoop, games and story books ................................ 5 years
```

OCCUPATIONS

Home Kindergarten

There are a number of books designed to teach mothers how to carry the Kindergarten occupations over into the home; but while such books may be helpful in a few cases, in most cases better occupations present themselves in the course of the day's work. The Kindergarten occupations themselves follow increasingly the order of domestic routine. For example, many children in the Kindergarten make mittens out of eiderdown flannel in the Fall, when their own mothers are knitting their mittens, and make little hoods either for themselves or for their dolls. At other periods they put up little glasses of preserves or jelly, and study the industry of the bees and the way they put up their tiny jars of jelly. Their attention is called also to the preparations that the squirrels and other animals make for winter, and to that of the trees and flowers. In other words, the occupations in the Kindergarten are designed to bring the children into conscious sympathy with the life of nature and of the home.

Kindergarten Methods

That mother who keeps this purpose in mind and applies it to the occupations that come up naturally in the course of a day's work, will thereby bring the Kindergarten spirit into her own home much more truly than if she invests in a number of perforated sewing cards and colored strips of paper for weaving. Not that there is any harm in these bits of apparatus, provided that the sewing cards are large and so perforated as not to task the eyes and young fingers of the sewer. But unless for some special purpose, such as the making of a Christmas or birthday gift, these devices are unnecessary and better left to the school, which has less richness of material at hand than has the home.

Helping Mother

In allowing the children to enter a workers into the full life of the home several good things are accomplished. (1) The eager interest of the developing mind is utilized to brighten those duties which are likely to remain permanent duties. Not does this observation apply only to girls. Domestic obligations are supposed to rest chiefly upon them, but the truth is that boys need to feel these obligations as keenly as the girls, if they are to grow into considerate and helpful husbands and fathers. The usual division of labor into forms falsely called masculine and feminine is, therefore, much to be deplored. Moreover, at an early age children are seldom sex-conscious, and any precocity in this direction is especially evil in its results; yet many mothers from the beginning make such a division between what they require of their boys and of their girls as to force this consciousness upon them. All kinds of work, then, should be allowed in the beginning, however it may differentiate later on, and little boys as well as little girls should be taught to take an interest in sewing, dish-washing, sweeping, dusting, and cooking—in all the forms of domestic activity.

This is so far recognized among educators that the most progressive primary schools now teach cooking to mixed classes of boys and girls, and also sewing. These activities are recognized as highly educational, being, as they are, interwoven with the history of the race and with its daily needs. When they are studied in their full sum of relationship, they increase the child's knowledge of both the past and the living world.

Teaching Mother

(2) Besides the deepening of the child's interest in that work which in some form or other he will have with him always, is the quickening of the mother's own interest in what may have come to seem to her mere daily drudgery. Any woman who undertakes to perform so simple an operation as dish-washing with the help of a bright happy child, asking sixteen questions to the minute, will find that common-place operation full of possibilities; and if she will answer all the questions she will probably find her knowledge strained to the breaking point, and will discover there is more to be known about dish-washing than she ever dreamed of before; while in cooking, if she will make an effort to look up the science, history, and ethics involved in the cooking and serving of a very simple meal, she will not be likely to regard the task as one beneath her, but rather as one beyond her. No one can so lead her away from false conventions and narrow prejudices as a little child whom she permits to help her and teach her.

The Love of Work

(3) The child's spontaneous joy in being active and in doing any service is being utilized, as it should be, in the performance of his daily duties. We have already referred to the fact that all children in the beginning love to work, and that there must be something the matter with our education since this love is so early lost and so seldom reacquired. If when young children wish to help mother they are almost invariably permitted to do so, and their efforts greeted lovingly, this delight in helpfulness will remain a blessing to them throughout life.

To Make "Helping" of Benefit

But in order to get these benefits from the domestic activities two or three simple rules must be observed. (1) Do not go silently about your work, expecting your child to be interested and to understand without being talked to. Play with him while you work with him, and see the realization of youthfulness that comes to yourself while you do it. Many tasks fit for childish hands are in their nature too monotonous for childish minds. Here your imagination must come into play to rouse and excite his activity. For instance, you are both shelling peas. When he begins to be tired you suggest to him, "Here is a cage full of birds, let us open the door for them;" or you may tell a story while you work, but it should be a story about that very activity, or the child will form the habit of dreaming and dawdling over his work. Such stories may be perfectly simple and even rather pointless and yet do good work; the whole object is to keep the child's fly-away imagination turned upon the work at hand, thus lending wings to his thought, and lightness to his fingers. Moreover, the mother who talks with her child while working is training in him the habit of bright unconscious conversation, thus giving him a most useful accomplishment. Making a game or a play out of the work is, of course, conducive to the same good results. When the story or the talk drags, the game with its greater dramatic power may be substituted.

Fatigue

(2) Children should neither be allowed to work to the point of fatigue nor to stop when they please. Fatigue, as our latest investigators in physiological psychology have conclusively proved, is productive of an actual poison in the blood and as such is peculiarly harmful to young children. But while work—or for that matter play either—must never be pushed past the point

of healthful fatigue, it may well be pushed past the point of spontaneous interest and desire: the child may be happily persuaded by various hidden means to do a little more than he is quite ready to do. By this device, which is one of the recognized devices of the Kindergarten, mothers increase by imperceptible degrees that power of attention which makes will power.

Willing Industry

(3) Set the example of willing industry. Neither let the child conceive of you as an impersonal necessary part of the household machinery, nor as an unwilling martyr to household necessities. Most mothers err in one or the other of these two directions, and many of them err in both: they either, (a) perform the innumerable services of the household so quietly and steadily that the child does not perceive the effort that the performance costs and, therefore, as far as his consciousness is concerned, is deprived of the force of his mother's example, or (b) they groan aloud over their burdens and make their daily martyrdom vocal. Either way is wrong, for it is a mistake not to let a child see that your steady performance of tasks, which cannot be always delightful, is a result of self-discipline; and it is equally a mistake to let him think that this discipline is one against which you rebel. For in reality you are so far from being unwilling to bind yourself in his service that if he needed it you would promptly double and quadruple your exertions. It is exactly what you do when he is sick or in danger; and if he dies the sorest ache of your heart is the ache of the love that can no longer be of service to the beloved.

Monotony

(4) Remember that monotony is the curse of labor for both child and adult, but that *monotony cannot exist where new intellectual insights are constantly being given*. Therefore, while the daily round of labor, shaped by the daily recurring demands for food, warmth, cleanliness, and sleep, goes on without much change, seize every opportunity to deepen the child's perception of the relation of this routine to the order of the larger world. For instance, if a new house is being built near by, visit it with the children, comparing it with your own house, figure out whether it is going to be easier to keep clean and to warm than your house is and why. If you need to call in the carpenter, the plumber, the paper-hanger, or the stoveman, try to have him come when the children are at home, and let them satisfy their

intense curiosity as to his work. This knowledge will sooner or later be of practical value, and it is immediately of spiritual value.

Beautiful Work

(5) Beautify the work as much as possible by letting the artistic sense have full play. This rule is so important that the attempt to establish it in the larger world outside of the home has given rise to the movement known as the arts and crafts movement, which has its rise in the perception that no great art can come into existence among us until the common things of daily living—the furniture, the books, the carpets, the chinaware—are made to express that creative joy in the maker which distinguishes an artistic product from an inartistic one. This creative joy, in howsoever small degree, may be present in most of the things that the child does. If he sets the table, he may set it beautifully, taking real pleasure in the coloring of the china and the shine of the silver and glass. He ought not to be permitted to set it untidily upon a soiled tablecloth.

The Right Spirit

(6) This is a negative rule, but perhaps the most important of all: DO NOT NAG. The child who is driven to his work and kept at it by means of a constant pressure of a stronger will upon his own, is deriving little, if any, benefit from it; and as you are not teaching him to work for the sake of his present usefulness, which is small at the best, but for the sake of his future development, you are more desirous that he should perform a single task in a day in the right spirit, than that he should run a dozen errands in the wrong spirit.

(7) Besides a regular time each day for the performance of his set share in the household work, give him warning before the arrival of that hour. Children have very incomplete notions of time; they become much absorbed in their own play; and therefore no child under nine or ten years of age should be expected to do a given thing at a given time without warning that the time is at hand.

"Busy Work"

Besides these occupations which are truly part of the business of life come any number of other occupations—a sort of a cross between real play and steady work, what teachers call "busy work"—and here the suggestions of the Kindergarten may be of practical value to the mother. For instance, weaving, already referred to, may keep an active child interested and quiet for considerable periods of time. Besides the regular weaving mats of paper, to be had from any Kindergarten supply store, wide grasses and rushes may be braided into mats, raffia and rattan may be woven into baskets, and strips of cloth woven into iron-holders. A visit to any neighboring Kindergarten will acquaint the mother with a number of useful, simple objects that can be woven by a child. Whatever he weaves or whatever he makes should be applied to some useful purpose, not merely thrown away; and while it is true that a conscientious desire to live up to this rule often results in a considerable clutter of flimsy and rather undesirable objects about the house, still, ways may be devised for slowly retiring the oldest of them from view, and disposing of others among patient relatives.

Sewing

Sewing is another occupation ranch used in the Kindergarten as well as in the home. Beginning with the simple stringing of large wooden beads upon shoe-strings, it passes on to sewing on buttons, and sewing doll clothes to the making of real clothing. This last in its simplest form can be begun sooner than most parents suppose, especially if the child is taught the use of the sewing machine. There is really no reason why a child, say six years old, should not learn to sew upon the machine. His interest in machinery is keen at this period, and two or three lessons are usually sufficient to teach him enough about the mechanism to keep him from injuring it. Once he has learned to sew upon the machine, he may be given sheets and towels to hem, and even sew up the seams of larger and more complex articles. He will soon be able to make aprons for himself and his sisters and mother. Toy sewing machines are now sold which are really useful playthings, and on which the child can manufacture a number of small articles. Those run by a treadle are preferable to those run by a hand crank, because they leave the child's hands free to guide the work.

Drawing Cutting Pasting

Drawing, painting, cutting and pasting are excellent occupations for children. A large black-board is a useful addition to the nursery furnishings, but the children should be required to wash it off with a damp cloth, instead of using the eraser furnished for the purpose, as the chalk dust gets into the room and fills the children's lungs. Plenty of soft pencils and crayons, also large sheets of inexpensive drawing paper, should be at hand upon a low table so that they can draw the large free outlines which best develop their skill, whenever the impulse moves them. If they have also blunt scissors for cutting all sorts of colored papers and a bottle of innocuous library paste, they will be able to amuse themselves at almost any time.

Painting

Some water colors are now made which are harmless for children so young that they are likely to put the paints in their mouths. Paints are on the whole less objectionable than colored chalks, because the crayons drop upon the floor and get trodden into the carpet. If children are properly clothed as they should be in simple washable garments, there is practically no difficulty connected with the free use of paints, and their educational value is, of course, very high.

TEST QUESTIONS

The following questions constitute the "written recitation" which the regular members of the A.S.H.E. answer in writing and send in for the correction and comment of the instructor. They are intended to emphasize and fix in the memory the most important points in the lesson.

STUDY OF CHILD LIFE

PART II

Read Carefully. In answering these questions you are earnestly requested *not* to answer according to the text-book where opinions are asked for, but to answer according to conviction. In all cases credit will be given for thought and original observation. Place your name and full address at the head of the paper; use your own words so that your instructor may be sure that you understand the subject.

1. State Fichte's doctrine of rights and show how it applies to child training. If possible, give an example from your own experience.

2. What is the aim of moral training?

3. What two sayings of Froebel most characteristically sum up his philosophy?

4. What is the value of play in education?

5. What are the natural playthings? Tell what, in your childhood, you got out of these things, or if you were kept away from them, what the prohibition meant to you.

6. What do you think about children's dancing? And acting?

7. Do you agree with those who think that the Kindergarten makes right doing too easy? State the reasons for your opinion.

8. What can you say of commands, reproofs, and rules?

9. Should you let the children help you about the house, even when they are so little as to be troublesome? Why? If they are unwilling to help, how do you induce them to help?

10. What would you suggest as regular duties for children of 4 to 5 years? Of 7 to 8 years?

11. Which do you consider the more important, the housework or the child?

12. Wherein may the mother learn from the child?

13. What is the difference between amusing children and playing with them? What is the proper method?

14. Mention some good rules in character building.

15. From your own experience as a child what can you say of teaching the mysteries of sex?

16. Are there any questions you would like to ask, or subjects which you wish to discuss in connection with this lesson?

Note.—After completing the test sign your full name.

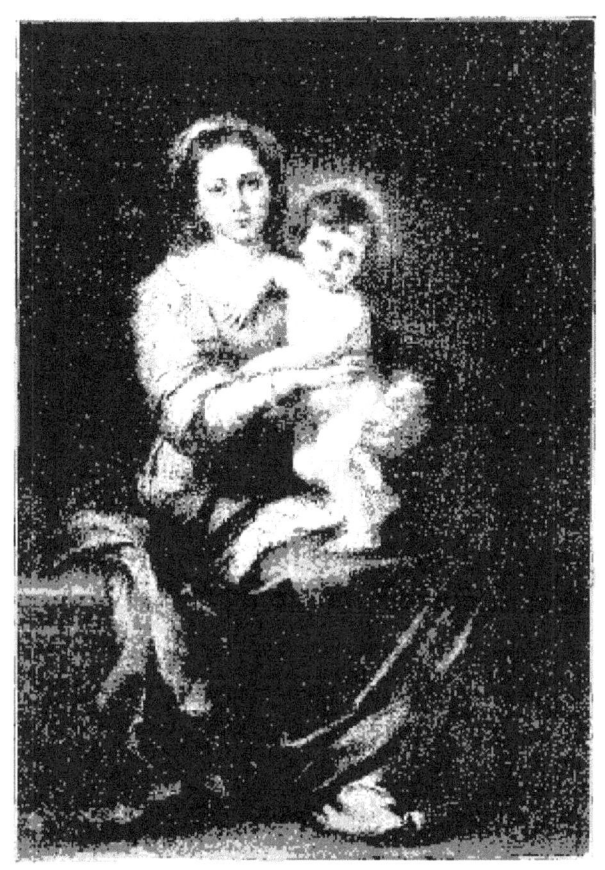

MADONNA AND CHILD
By Murillo, Spanish painter of the seventeenth century

STUDY OF CHILD LIFE

PART III

ART AND LITERATURE IN CHILD LIFE

The influence of art upon the life of a young child is difficult of measurement. It may freely be said, however, that there is little or no danger in exaggerating its influence, and considerable danger in underrating it. It is difficult of measurement because the influence is largely an unconscious one. Indeed, it may be questioned whether that form of art which gives him the most conscious and outspoken pleasure is the form that in reality is the most beneficial; for, unquestionably, he will get great satisfaction from circus posters, and the poorly printed, abominably illustrated cheap picture-books afford him undeniable joy. He is far less likely to be expressive of his pleasure in a sun-shiny nursery, whose walls, rugs, white beds, and sun-shiny windows are all well designed and well adapted to his needs. Nevertheless, in the end the influence of this room is likely to be the greater influence and to permanently shape his ideas of the beautiful; while he is entirely certain, if allowed to develop artistically at all, to grow past the circus poster period.

This fact—the fact that the highest influence of art is a secret influence, exercised not only by those decorations and pictures which flaunt themselves for the purpose, but also by those quiet, necessary, every-day things, which nevertheless may most truly express the art spirit—this fact makes it difficult to tell what art and what kind of art is really influencing the child, and whether it is influencing him in the right directions.

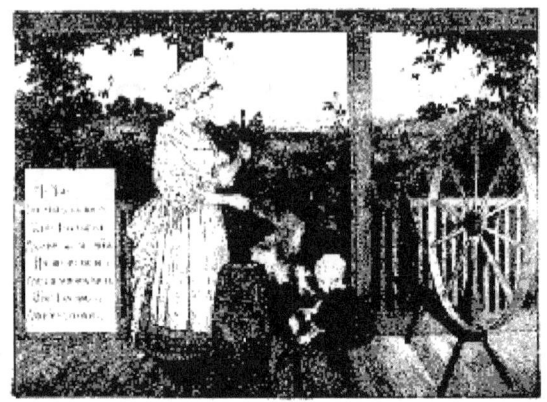
"Be Mary"

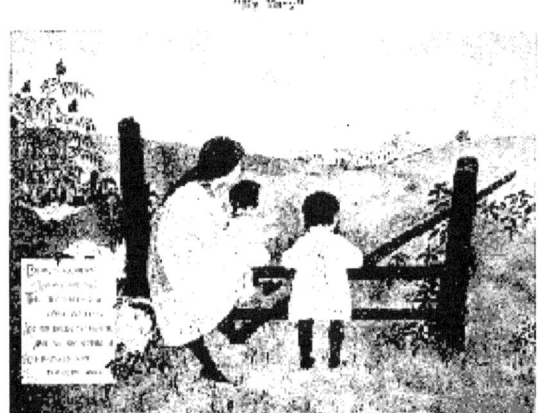
"Bow Wow Wow"
PERKINS' PICTURES

Color

Until he is three years old, for example, and often until he is past that age, he is unable to distinguish clearly between green, gray and blue; and hence these cool colors in the decorations around him, or in his pictures, have practically no meaning for him. He has a right, one might suppose, to the gratification of his love for clear reds and yellows, for the sharp, well-defined lines and flat surfaces, whose meaning is plain to his groping little mind. Some of the best illustrators of children's books have seemed to recognize this. For example, Boutet de Monvil in his admirable illustrations of Joan of Arc meets these requirements perfectly, and yet in a manner which must satisfy any adult lover of good art. The Caldecott picture books, and Walter Crane's are also good in this respect, and the Perkins pictures issued by the Prang Educational Co. have gained a just recognition as excellent pictures for hanging on the nursery wall. Many of the illustrations in color in the standard magazines are well worth cutting out, mounting and framing. This is especially true of Howard Pyle's work and that of Elizabeth Shippen Green.

Classic Art

Since photogravures and photographs of the masterpieces can be had in this country very inexpensively, there is no reason why children should not be made acquainted at an early age with the art classics, but there is danger in giving too much space to black and white, especially in the nursery where the children live. Their natural love of color should be appealed to do deepen their interest in really good pictures.

Nevertheless, it is a matter of considerable difficulty still to find colored pictures which are inexpensive and yet really good. The Detaille prints, while not yet cheap, are not expensive either, and are excellent for this purpose; but the insipid little pictures of fairies, flowers, and birds may be really harmful, as helping to form in the young child's mind too low an ideal of beauty—of cultivating in him what someone has called "the lust of the eye."

Plastic Art

What holds true of the pictorial art holds equally true of the plastic art. As Prof. Veblin of the University of Chicago has scathingly declared, our ideals of the beautiful are so mingled with worship of expense that few of us can see the genuine beauty in any object apart from its expensiveness. For this reason as well as, perhaps, because of a remnant of barbarism in us, we love gold and glitter, and a great deal of elaboration in our vases, and are far from being over-critical of any piece of statuary which costs a respectable sum.

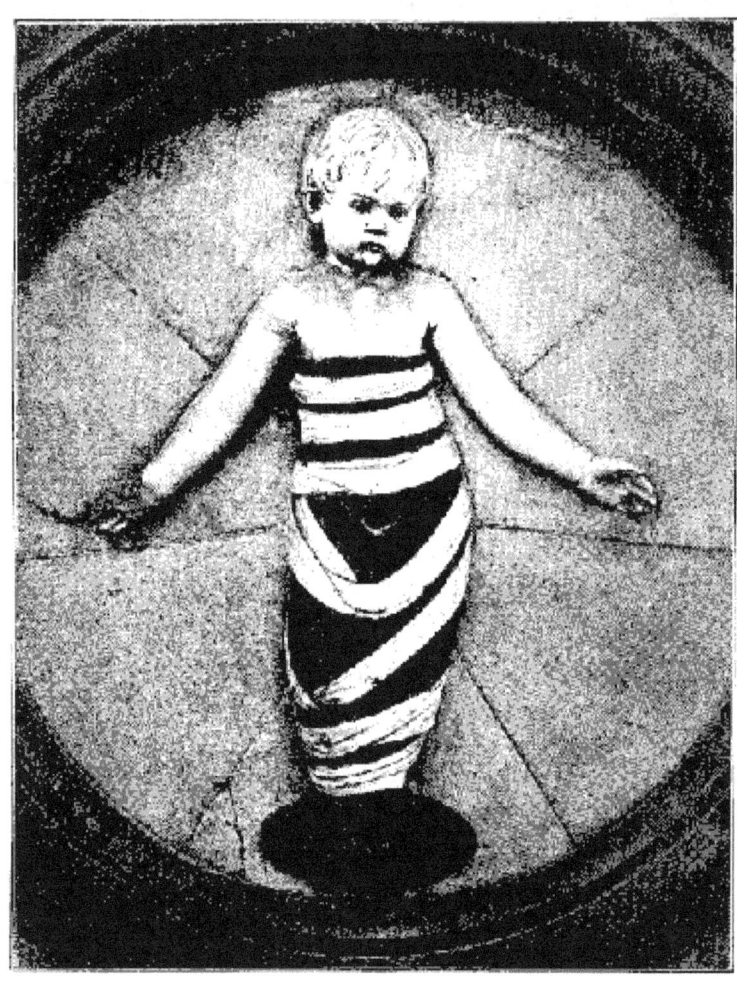

RELIEF MEDALLION
By Andrea della Robbia, in Foundling Hospital, Florence.

A certain appreciation, however, of the real value of a good plaster-cast has been gaining among us of late years, and many public schools, especially in the large cities, have been establishing standards of good taste in this respect. Good casts and bas-relief, decorate their halls and class-rooms. There are few homes that cannot afford to follow their example. But in buying these things be not misled by sales and advertised bargains. It is more than seldom that the placques, casts, and vases thus obtained are such as could have any valuable influence whatever upon the young lives with which they are brought in contact. Meretricious and showy ornaments, designed to look as if they cost more than they really do, have no business in the sincere home where the children are being sincerely educated.

Music

The same general laws apply to music. No art has a greater and more insinuating influence. The very songs with which the mother sings the baby to sleep have an occult influence which is later revealed and made plain. Such songs, then, should be simple. They may be nothing but improvisations, the mother's mind and heart making music, but they should not be melodramatic songs of the music-hall order. No such mawkish sentimentalism as that shown in "The Gypsy's Warning," for example, or other songs which belong to the cheap theater should have a place in the holy of holies—that inmost self of the child—which responds to music.

The simple folk-songs of all nations, Eleanor Smith's and most of Mrs. Gaynor's songs, already mentioned, and the songs collected by Reinecke, called "Fifty Children's Songs," are excellent for this purpose. The old-fashioned nonsense songs, such as "Billy Boy," "Mary had a Little Lamb" and "Hey Diddle Diddle, the Cat and the Fiddle," may also have a pleasant and harmless place of their own.

Instrumental music should be on the same general order, not loud and showy, but clear, simple, sweet, and free from startling effects. Dashing pieces, rag-time pieces, marches, two-steps, and familiar tunes with variations, instead of bringing about a spirit of gentleness and harmony, actually tend to produce self-assertiveness and quarrelsomeness. Let any mother who does not believe this try the effort of an hour of the one kind of music on one evening, and an hour of the other kind on another evening. The difference will be immediately apparent.

The Drama

The influence of the drama must not be forgotten. This form of art, fallen so low among us since the time of the Puritans that it can scarcely be called an art at all, is, nevertheless, the art which perhaps above all others has an immediate and yet lasting influence. Children are themselves instinctively dramatic. They like to compose and act out all sorts of dramas of their own, from playing house (which is nothing but a drama prolonged from day to day), to such dramatic games as Statue-posing and Dumb Crambo. All children like to dress up, to wear masks, and to imitate the peculiarities of persons about them; to try on, as it were, the world as they see it, and discover thereby how the actors in it feel. Goethe's Wilhelm Meister has already been referred to. In this—his great book on education—he practically bases all education upon the drama, and even throws the treatise itself into dramatic form.

This does not mean, however, that all children should be permitted to go to the theater as freely as they like. No; the plays which they compose and act for themselves have a far higher value educationally than most of the spectacular presentations of the old fairy tales with which they are usually regaled, and certainly more than the sensational melodramas which give them false ideas of art and morality. They should go sometimes to the theater to see really good and simple plays, but they should be oftener encouraged to get up for themselves plays at home. If, as they grow older, they are helped to think out their costumes with something of historical accuracy, to be true to the spirit and scenery of the times in which the representations are laid, the activity can be made to increase in value to them as the years go by. There is no other art, perhaps, by which the child so intimately links the world spirit with his own spirit. It is for this reason that the School of Education in the University of Chicago is equipped with small theaters in which the children act.

Literature

As for the art of literature, not all children love reading, perhaps, but certainly all children love to hear stories told, and the skilful mother will direct this spontaneous affection into a love for reading. No other single love, except perhaps the love of nature, so emancipates the child from the thrall of circumstances. If he can escape from the small ills of life into fairy-land merely by opening the covers of a book, be sure that these ills will not have power to crush him, unless they be very great ills indeed.

Fairy Tales

There are those who still believe that fairy-tales and fiction of all sorts are nothing but lies. Poor souls, with their faces against the stone wall of hard facts, they can never look up into the sky and see the winged and beautiful thoughts freely disporting there. They make no distinction between truth and fact, yet truth is of the spirit and fact of the flesh; and truth, because it is of the spirit, may appear under many forms, even under the form of play. All rightly told and rightly conceived fairy-tales are true just as a good picture is true. The painter uses oil, turpentine, and pigment to represent the wool of a sheep, the water of a pond, the green spears of grass. Some literal-minded person might say that he was lying because he pretended that his little square of canvas truthfully represented grazing sheep at the brookside, but most of us recognize that he is really telling the truth only in another than an every day form. In the same way the writer of fairy-tales tells the truth, using the pigments of the imagination.

If children ask whether a given story is true or not, answer without hesitation, "yes." It is true, but it is a fairy kind of truth; it is inside truth. There is magic in it and a mystery. The child who is never allowed to read fairy tales, the man or the woman who prefers the newspaper to a good book of fiction, misses much in life. It is not only that the imagination—the divinest quality of man, because the quality that makes man in his degree a creator—does not receive culture, and that he misses the indescribable intellectual ecstasy that comes only with the setting free of the wings of the mind, but that also he is inevitably shorn of his sympathy and shut up to a narrow circle of interests.

Imagination and Sympathy

For sympathy, above all moral qualities, is dependent upon imagination. If you cannot imagine how you would feel under your neighbor's conditions, you cannot deeply sympathize with him. The person of unimaginative mind sympathizes only with those whose experience and habits are similar to his own. He never escapes from the narrow circle of his own personality. But the man whose imagination has been kept flexible and ready from earliest childhood has within him the power of sympathizing with whatever is human—yes! even with creatures and things below the human level. Without imagination, therefore, it is not possible for a man to be a great scientist, for science demands sympathy with processes and objects which are not yet human. It is not possible, obviously, for him to be a great artist of any kind, for all art is interpretation of the world by means of the imagination. It is not possible for him, even, to be a good man in any broad sense, for the man whose sympathies are narrow is often found to be guilty of injustice toward those who lie outside the pale of those sympathies.

By all means, then, encourage the love of reading in your children, and get them the best of story-books to read, and subscribe to the best magazines. Read with them. Let some reading enter into every day's life; talk over what has been read at the dinner-table, and so avoid harmful personalities and disagreeable criticisms.

Books

As to the books to choose, choose the best. Generally speaking, the best are those that have some dignity of age upon them. As in music you chose the folksongs, so in children's literature also choose the old fashioned fairy stories, such as those collected by the Brothers Grimm and by Andrew Lang. Hans Christian Andersen's Fairy Stories of course are classics. Hawthorne's Tanglewood Tales give excellent suggestions as to the right use to be made of the old mythologies. Many of the supplementary readers now being so widely used in the public schools are good, simple versions of these old stories which helped to make the world what it should be. For the rest there are two standard children's magazines which help to form a good taste in literature and which are continually suggestive of the right sort of reading material. These are The Youth's Companion and St. Nicholas.

Nature Study

Finally, all appreciation of literature and art depends upon a love of and some knowledge of nature. Fairy stories and mythology especially are so dependent upon nature for their inner meaning and significance as scarcely to be intelligible without some knowledge of natural processes and laws. Of course, it is true that art in its turn idealizes nature and fills her beautiful form with a beautiful soul; so that the child who is being developed on all sides needs to take his books and his pictures out of doors in order to get the full good of them.

Art and Nature

No amount of music, art, and literature can make up for the free life in the fields and under the sky which all these arts describe and interpret. If he should be so unhappy as to have to choose between nature and art, it would be better for him to choose nature, because then, perhaps, art might be born in his own soul. But there is happily no need for such a painful choice. He can sing his little song out of doors with the birds and notice how they join in the chorus. He can paint evening sunsets with the pine-trees against it far better out of doors than indoors with copy perched before him. He can look down the aisles of the real woods to watch for the enchanted princess, or for the chivalrous knight whose story he is reading. Art and nature belong together in the unified soul of the child. Well for him and for the world in which he lives if they are never divorced, but he goes on to the end loving them both and seeing them both as one.

CHILDREN'S ASSOCIATES.

If the child was intended to grow into a man of family, merely, family training might be sufficient for him, but since he must grow into a member of society, social training is as necessary for him as family training. Failure to recognize this truth is at the bottom of the current misconceptions of the Kindergarten. There are still thousands of persons who suppose it is only a superior sort of day-nursery where children may be safely kept and innocently employed while the mother gets the housework done.

The Kindergarten

While this might be a laudable enough function to perform, it is by no means the function of the Kindergarten. This method of instruction aims at much more. It aims to lay foundations for a complete later education, and especially to make firm in the child those virtues and aptitudes which, when they are held by the majority of men, constitute the safety and welfare of society. For this reason no home, however well ordered, can supply to the child what the Kindergarten supplies. For the home is necessarily limited to the members of one family, while the Kindergarten, on the contrary, makes plain to the child the claims upon him of society not made up of his kinsfolk. It is the wide world in miniature, and if it is a properly organized Kindergarten, it will contain within itself a wide variety of children—children of wealth and of poverty, of ignorance and of gentle breeding—and will bring them all under one just rule. For only by this commingling of many characters upon a common level and under the strict reign of justice can the child be fitted practically, and by means of a series of progressive experiments, for citizenship in a genuine democracy.

Exclusive Associates

Parents sometimes so far miss the aim of the Kindergarten as to desire that instead of such a commingling there shall be a narrow limit set; that in the Kindergarten shall be only such children as the child is accustomed to associate with. But if the Kindergarten acceded to this demand, as it seldom does, it would lose much of its usefulness, for every one knows that children cannot be permanently sheltered from contact with the outside world, nor can they be always reared in an atmosphere of exclusiveness. A wisdom greater than the mother's has ordered that no child shall be so narrowly nourished. If he has any freedom whatever, any naturalness of life, he must and will enlarge his circle of acquaintances beyond the limit of his mother's calling list.

Indeed, even those Kindergartens which are professedly exclusive, and which confine their ministrations to the children of one particular neighborhood, are obliged by the nature of things to contain nascent individualities of almost every type. For no neighborhood, however equal in wealth and fashion, ever produced children of an unvarying quality. In any circle, no matter how exclusive, there are mischievous children, children who use bad language, children who have sly, mean tricks, children who do not speak the truth, and who are in other ways quite as undesirable as the children of the poor and ignorant. It is often asserted, indeed, that the children of exclusive neighborhoods very often show more varieties of badness than the children of the open street. The records of the private Kindergarten as compared with the public Kindergarten amply prove this statement.

Evil Example

Since, then, whether you confine your child to the limits of your own circle or not, you cannot successfully keep him from playing with children who are more or less objectionable, what are you going to do to keep him from the harm of such association? You have to make him strong enough to withstand temptation and resist the force of evil example. Of course, he must have as little of the wrong example, especially in his younger and tenderer years, as can be managed without too greatly checking his activity and curtailing his freedom. Yet after all he is to be taught a positive and not a negative righteousness, and if his home training is not sufficient to enable him to stand against a certain downward pull from the outside, there is something the matter with it.

While he must not be strained too hard, nor too constantly associate with children whose manners put his manners to the test, still he ought by degrees, almost imperceptibly, to be accustomed to holding to the truth, to that which is found good, no matter whether his associates find it desirable or not.

Social Training

A good Kindergarten is a mother's best help in this endeavor, for there her child meets with all sorts of other children. The very influence of the place, and the ever-ready help of the teacher are on his side. Every effort he makes to do right is met and welcomed. In every stand that he takes against temptation, he is unobtrusively reinforced. Moreover, the wrong-doing of his comrades is never allowed to retain the attractive glitter that it sometimes acquires on the play-ground. It is promptly held up to general obloquy, and the good child finds to his surprise that he is not the only one who thinks that teasing, for example, is mean and selfish and that a violent temper is ugly.

Responsibility to Society

Moreover, in the Kindergarten the sense of social responsibility is borne in upon him. Perhaps it comes to him first when he is chosen to lead the march and finds that he must be careful not to squeeze through too narrow places, lest someone get into trouble. In dealing out pencils, worsted, and other materials he must be careful to show strict impartiality, and give no preference to his own personal friends. In a hundred small ways he is helped to regulate his own conduct, so that it may conduce to the welfare of the whole school.

Where there are no Kindergartens, the task becomes a more difficult one for the mother, for it becomes necessary, then, that she herself should undertake the social training of her child, and this means that she must know his playmates, not only through his report of them, but through her own observation of them, and that they must be sufficiently at home with her to betray their true characters in her presence. And this means, of course, that she must become her child's playmate. There are few women who think that they have time for this, but there are also few who would not be benefited by it. If anywhere there is a fountain of youth, it gushes up invisibly wherever playing children are, and she who plays with them gets sprinkled by it.

Sharing the Child's Play

If there be no time during the busy day when she can justly enter into the children's free play, at least there is a little while in the late afternoon or in the early evening when she can do so, if she will. An hour or two a week spent in active association with children at their games will make her intimately acquainted with all their playmates, and, moreover, constitute her a power of first magnitude among them. Her motherhood thus extends itself, and she blesses not only her own children, but all those who come near her children. In this respect no Kindergarten can take the place of the mother's own companionship with the child in his social life.

The Children's Hour

In an ideal condition the child has his Kindergarten in the morning; his quiet hours, one of them entirely solitary, in the afternoon; his social time, when he, his brothers and sisters and mother, are joined with the other children and mothers in the neighborhood, in the late afternoon, and his family time, with both father and mother, in the evening before going to bed.

In thus sharing her child's social life the mother admits the claim upon her of social responsibility; she sees that her duty is not to her own home alone, but to the other homes with which hers is linked—not to her own child alone, but to all children whose lives touch her child's life. Her own nature widens with the perception, and she enhances her direct teaching with the force of a beautiful example.

STUDIES AND ACCOMPLISHMENTS

Abstract Studies

There may easily be too many studies and too many accomplishments in the life of any child. As our schools are constituted there are certainly too many studies of the wrong kind being carried on every day. But there are also too few studies of the right kind. In one of our large cities a test was once made as to how much the children who left school at the fifth grade, as 70 per cent of them do, had actually learned in a way that would be of practical value to them, and the results were most discouraging. These city children who could recite their tables of measurements with glibness, and who performed with a fair degree of success several hundred examples dealing with units of measure, could not tell whether their school-room floor contained one acre or two hundred and forty! None of them suspected that it contained less than an acre. Although they could bound the States of the Union, and give the principal exports and imports, they knew next to nothing of their own city and of its actual relation to the countries which they studied in their geography lessons. The teachers, in explanation, laid much of the blame for this state of affairs upon the parents, saying that they took but little interest in their children's studies, and never attempted to link them to the things of every-day life. But while this claim might be justified to some extent, it was by no means sufficient to cover the facts of the case. The truth is, it was quite as much the teachers' duty to link these abstract studies with concrete facts, as it was the parents'.

Dead Knowledge

Such an experience, however, suggests the manner in which parents can best help on the work of children in school. So long as these studies are still taught in the dead, monotonous way common to text-books, children will be racked nervously, and not benefited mentally in the effort to master them. Fathers and mothers who by the exercise of some ingenuity manage to show the child that his arithmetical knowledge is of actual help in solving the questions of every-day life; that his history has bearings upon the progress of events around him, and that his geography relates to actual places which, perhaps, father and mother may have seen, or which their books tell about—such fathers and mothers will make their children's school work easier, at the same time that they increase the sum of their children's knowledge. It is dead knowledge only—knowledge wrenched from its living content—that is difficult of digestion.

The New Education

It is natural for a young mind to like to learn, as it is for a healthy stomach to be supplied with food; but knowledge, like the food, must be fit for the use that is to be made of it and for the organ that is to receive it; and the brain, like the stomach, has a signal which it flies to show whether the food is what it wants or not. The brain exhibits interest exactly as the stomach exhibits appetite. The object of scientific education is to discover what the spontaneous, universal interest of children of certain ages is, and to meet that interest with the fullest possible supply of knowledge in every conceivable form.

Scientific education does not depend upon text-books or upon merely verbal explanations, but gets the idea home to the child by the means of a varied appeal to all the senses and sensibilities. For this reason the most advanced schools have many more studies and what are commonly called accomplishments than the public or parochial schools. That is, they add to the three r's—reading, 'riting and 'rithmetic—drawing, modeling, painting, manual training, physical culture, dramatic representation, music, field trips, and laboratory work.

Correlation of Studies

Yet this apparently great increase of subjects in the number of studies actually lessens the amount of work required of the child, because all these different activities, by means of what is called correlation, are brought to bear upon the same subject. For example, the class which goes out for a field trip to visit a near-by brook sees the water actually at work, cutting its way to the river, and thence to the sea. They measure its force and note its effects; they make a water-color sketch of some curve of it; they notice what birds and insects are about; what flowers grow there; what indications there may be of burrowing animals. When they get back to school they model, perhaps, some bird that they have noticed; or in the geographical laboratory, with streams of water try to reproduce in miniature the action of the brook upon the soil through which it flows.

For their arithmetic lesson they estimate the number of years the brook must have been flowing to have cut its valley to its present depth. They make a full report and description of their day's work for their reading and writing lesson. They have thus gained an immense amount of information, and have done a great deal of hard work; but instead of being nervously exhausted, they are bright and exhilarated. Such fatigue as they know is wholesome and fits them for a sound night's sleep.

Home Expedients

When it is impossible to send the child to such a school as this, something may be done by supplementing the ordinary school by some of these procedures. The clay jar, the crayons, and the paints have already been suggested, and with the parents' interest in the child's studies, helping him to model and paint things which he studies at school, he will instantly show the good effect of the home training and encouragement. As for field trips, the regular Sunday walk, or evening stroll, may be made to take its place. If you think that you do not know enough to teach your child on these walks, give him then the privilege of teaching you. He will work the harder in order to rise to the occasion.

Physical Culture

As for physical culture, if your school is without it, your barn, your parlor, and your lawn may supply it in some sort. In the barn may be a trapeze; there is already the ladder and the hay-loft; on the lawn may be a swing, trees to climb, and the tennis court. In your parlor may be a little home dancing school, where for a half an hour or so, the children march, skip, or two-step to music of your making. In the wood shed may be a carpenter's bench with real tools, where he may work and get some of the good of manual training.

Showy Accomplishments

Accomplishments, meaning thereby showy things that children do for the edification of guests, are of doubtful value. It is pleasant, of course, to have your little girl play a piece or two on the piano to entertain your visitors, but it is not nearly so important as health and strength, and a cheerful temper. Sometimes all three of these are sacrificed to the two or three hours' practice a day. Often, too, this extra work after school hours—work full as monotonous and nervous and uninteresting as the school work itself—is just what is needed to transform a healthy young girl into a nervous invalid. This is especially true, if she undertakes, as she usually does, to study music when she is about thirteen years old—the very time when, if wise physicians could regulate affairs to their liking, she would be taken out of school altogether and required to do nothing more than a little light housework every day.

Natural Talent

Of course, if she is naturally musical some kind of help and sympathy must be given her in her attempt to master the piano or violin or to manage her own voice. But while she should be allowed to learn as much as her unurged energies permit her to learn, she should not be required to practice more than a very small amount, say half an hour a day. The bulk of her musical education should be acquired in the vacation time, when she can give two hours a day without overstraining.

The same general rules hold good of dancing, painting, the acquirements of foreign languages, a special course of reading, or any other work undertaken in addition to the regular school work. This latter, as it is now constituted, is quite as severe a nervous and intellectual strain as most young people can undergo with safety.

"Enthusiasms"

There is one characteristic in young people which needs to be noted in this connection:—the desire to take up some form of work, to strive with it furiously for a brief while, to drop it unfinished; take up another with equal eagerness, drop that in turn and go on to a third. This performance is peculiarly irritating to all systematic and ambitious parents. Sometimes they rigidly insist that each task shall be finished before a new one is assumed. But in reality, is this necessary? It seems to be as natural for a young mind to set eagerly to work for a short time at each new bit of knowledge, as it is for a nursing child to require refreshments every two or three hours. It is an adult trait to stick to a task, even though a very long one, until it is accomplished. The youthful trait is to take kindly to a clutter of unfinished tasks.

The youthful consciousness is of a world full of jostling interests. Why not let the children alone, and allow them to spring lightly from one enthusiasm to another? Of course you will help them to finish, either at the first sitting or at the second or at the third, the task that was undertaken when that particular enthusiasm was at its height. The drawing which has remained on the easel during the foot-ball season may be suggestively brought to notice again in the quiet times between Thanksgiving and Christmas. The boat begun last summer may well be finished in the days of the succeeding Spring when all the earth is full of the sound of running water. Thus each task, though not completed at once, gets done in the end; and the youthful capacity for many sympathies and many desires has not been narrowed.

Parental Vanity

Such a line of conduct presupposes, of course, that the parent considers only the child's best welfare, and not his own parental vanity. He is not desirous that his son shall do anything so well as to attract the attention and admiration of the neighbors. He is desirous merely that the boy shall grow up wholesomely and happily, showing such superiority as there may be in him when the fitting time and opportunity present themselves. He will not attempt to make a musician of an unmusical child, nor a mechanic of an artistic child. He will not object to the brilliant and impractical dreams of the young inventor, but will help to make them practicable; and though he may squirm at some of the investigations of the budding scientist, he will not forbid them.

Development of Intellect

For such a parent recognizes that the important thing, educationally, is to secure the reaction of expression upon thought and feeling. That is, he is not trying to secure at this time—at any time during youth—perfect expression of any thought or feeling, but only to deepen feeling and clarify thought by encouraging all attempts at expression. He does not wish his child to make a finished picture or a perfect statue, but to acquire a greater sensitiveness to color and form by each attempt to express that color and form which he already knows. Thus whatever studies and accomplishments his child may be in the act of acquiring are seen to be nothing as acquisitions, but the child himself is seen to be growing stage by stage within the clumsy scaffolding.

FINANCIAL TRAINING

The financial training of children ought really to be considered under the head of moral training, but in some respects it can come equally well under the head of intellectual training; for to spend money well requires both self-control and intelligence. Some persons seem to think that all that a child can be taught in this regard is to save money, and they meet the situation by purchasing various shapes and styles of savings banks. But it is entirely possible to teach the child too thoroughly in this respect and to make him so fond of his jingling pennies safe within a yellow crockery pig or iron cupolaed mansion that be will not spend them for any object, however laudable. Others evade the issue as long as possible by giving the child no money at all; while most of us pursue an uncertain and wabbly course, sometimes giving money, sometimes withholding it, sometimes exhorting the child to spend, and sometimes to save.

Regular Allowance

In truth spending wisely is a difficult problem. As a rule the child may safely be induced to lay by for a season and then encouraged to spend for some generous purpose. Christmas and other festivals offer excellent opportunities for proper disbursement of the hoarded funds. These may be supposed to have accumulated from irregular gifts; but as the child grows older he should come into receipt of a regular definite allowance, perhaps conditioned upon his performance of some stated duty. A certain part of his allowance he may he permitted to spend upon such frivolities as are naturally dear to his young heart; another part of it he should be encouraged —not commanded—to put aside for larger purposes.

The giving of this allowance must not be confused with the pernicious habit of bribing the child to the performance of those little daily courtesies and duties which he ought to be willing to perform out of love and a sense of right. A certain part of his daily work, such as seeing that the match-boxes all over the house are filled, or some similar share of the general labor of the household, may be regarded as that for which he is paid wages; and any extra task which does not justly belong to him, he may sometimes be paid for performing; but not always. For instance, he ought to be willing to run to the grocery for mother without demanding that he be paid a penny for the job; yet sometimes the penny may be forthcoming. The point is that he should be ready to work, even to work hard, without pay, and yet that he should never feel that his mother withholds pay from him when she can give it and he receive it without injury.

Spending Foolishly

When the money is once his, he should be allowed to feel the full happiness and responsibility of possession, and if he insists upon spending it foolishly, should be allowed to do it and to suffer to the full the uncomfortable consequences. If, on the contrary, he will not spend it at all, his mother must use every means in her power to lessen the desire for ownership and to increase his love for others and his eagerness to please them.

As judgment develops the allowance may well be increased to provide for necessities in the way of incidentals and clothing until at the "age of discretion" he is in full charge of the funds for his personal expenses. He should be encouraged to apply his knowledge of commercial arithmetic in the keeping of personal accounts.

Experience in spending a fixed amount of money is especially needful for the daughters. Most young men have the value of money and financial responsibility forced upon them in the natural course of events, but too often the young wife has not had the training qualifying her for the equal financial partnership which should exist in the ideal marriage.

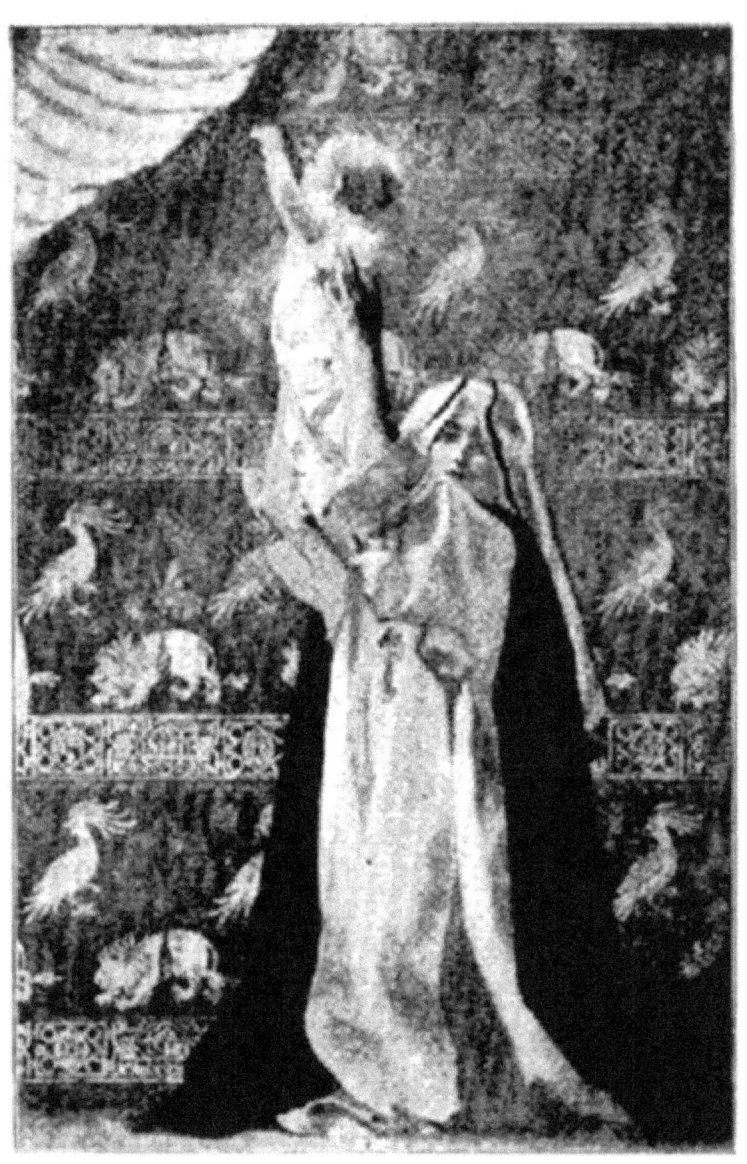

THE INFANT GALAHAD—FIRST SIGHT OF THE GRAIL.
From the mural paintings by Edwin A. Abbey in the
Boston Public Library

RELIGIOUS TRAINING

Sunday School Teachers

If the common school is not sufficient for the secular education of the child, certainly the Sunday School is not sufficient for his religious education. In the common schools the teachers are more or less trained for their work. It is a life occupation with them; by means of it they earn their living, and their daily success with their pupils marks their rate of progress toward higher fields of endeavor. Nothing of this sort is true in the Sunday School. While occasionally it happens that a day school teacher becomes a Sunday School teacher, this is seldom true, for most teachers who teach during the week feel that they need the Sunday for rest; and while some Sunday School teachers betray a commendable earnestness and zeal for their work, and associations and conventions have latterly added somewhat to the joint effort to better the conditions, still it remains true that the teaching in the Sunday Schools is far below the pedagogic level of the common schools. Yet the subject which is dealt with in the Sunday Schools, instead of being of less importance than that dealt with in the common schools, is of pre-eminently greater importance. Because of its subtlety, its intimacy with the hidden springs of conduct, it calls for the exercise of the very highest teaching skill.

Some sort of recognition of these two facts—that Sunday School teachers are in most cases very inadequately trained for their work, and that the work itself is of great importance, and of equally great difficulty—has led to the issuing of many quarterlies, International Lesson Leaflets, and other Sunday School aids. Necessary as such help may be under present conditions, they cannot possibly meet the many difficulties of the case. If the central committees, who issue these leaflets, were composed wholly of the wisest men and women on earth, it would still be impossible for them to give lessons to the millions of children in their various denominations which should meet the personal needs, and daily interests of these young people.

Sunday School Training

As a consequence, Sunday School teaching is and must be largely theoretical and still more largely exegetical, and with neither theory nor exegesis is the young mind of the developing child very much concerned. What he needs is not the historical side of religion or of that great body of religious literature which we call the Bible, but a living faith which links all that was taught by the prophets and apostles, centuries ago, with what is happening in the child's own town and family at that very moment. It is a wide gap to bridge, and it cannot be bridged by a semi-historical review backed by picture cards, golden texts, and stars for good behavior. These things are merely the marks of an endeavor to fitly accomplish a great task, an endeavor almost absurdly out of proportion to this aim, rendered significant, however, because it is the earnest of a great faith and a great hope.

So far as Sunday Schools help children, it is because of this spirit of faithfulness, and not because of the form which it has assumed.

In choosing, then, whether you shall send your child to a Sunday School, choose by the presence or absence of this spirit. If you know the teachers of the Sunday School to be earnest, loving, and devoted, you may with safety assume that their personal influence will make up for what is archaic in their method of teaching. Where the spirit is present only in a few, or where it manifests itself only occasionally, as at seasons of revival, you may well hesitate to let your child attend. A great improvement would come about if parents would show a greater interest and encourage proper teachers to take charge of classes. It is a thankless task at present.

Theory Not Practice

There is one great danger in the teaching of any Sunday School—one which the best of them cannot wholly escape—and that is, that, in the very nature of things, they teach theory and not practice. Harmful as this may be, indeed as it surely is in adult life, it does not begin to be so harmful as it does in youth, for the young child, as we have seen, is and should remain a unit in consciousness. His life, his intellect, and his will are one—an undivided trinity. The divorce of these three is at any time a regrettable occurrence; the divorce of them in early life is an almost irreparable disaster.

Useless Truths

The current theory is that children will learn many truths in the Sunday School which they will not put into practice then, perhaps, but which they will find useful in later life. This fallacy underlies, of course, almost all conventional education and has only been overthrown by the dictum of modern psychology, that there is but small storage accommodation in the brain for facts which have no immediate relation to life. What may be termed the saturating power of the brain is limited, and after it has soaked up a rather small number of truths, it can contain no more until it has in some way disposed of those that it still has—either by making them part of its own living structure, which is done only by making immediate application of them; or by dropping them below the threshold of consciousness, that is, in common language, forgetting them. Moreover, the brain may form the habit of easily dropping all that relates to a given subject into the limbo where unused things lie disregarded, and when this becomes the habitual method of disposing of religious instruction, the results are particularly deplorable.

The Mother as Teacher

Feeble as her own knowledge may be, a mother has certain advantages as a teacher of her children over any but the exceptional Sunday school teacher. For, first, she knows the children, and, knowing them, knows their needs. Secondly, she knows their daily lives and continually during the week can point out wherein they fail to live up to their Sunday's lesson. And again and most important, she loves them tenderly, and from love flows wisdom. Usually the mother gives her own children a love far beyond that given by anyone else, and this deeper love sharpens her intellectual faculties and makes her both a keen observer and a good tactician. Giving her children some simple lesson on Sunday afternoon, she finds a hundred opportunities to make the lesson living and vital to them during the succeeding week.

Religious Enthusiasm

In the early years of the child's life, the mother is usually the one to decide whether he shall attend Sunday School or not, but as he approaches adolescence he is likely to take the matter in his own hands, and if it happens that some revivalist or a new stirring preacher comes in contact with his life at this time, he is very likely to be swept off his feet with a sudden zeal of religious enthusiasm, which his mother fears to check. The reports of memberships, baptisms, etc., show that a large number become converted and join the church during adolescence. While this does not in the least argue that the conclusions that they reach at that time are therefore unsound—for adolescence is not a disease, nor a form of insanity, but a normal, if excitable, condition—still it does prove, when coupled with the further fact that in adult life these young converts often relapse into their previous condition, that a more lasting basis for religion must be found than the emotional intensity of this period of life. A religion to be lasting must be coldly reaffirmed by the intellect: the dictum of the heart alone is not sufficient. Religious enthusiasm, like all other forms of enthusiasm, tends of itself to bring about the opposite condition, and to be succeeded by fits of despondency and bitterness as intense and severe as the enthusiasm itself was brilliant and ecstatic. The history of all great religious leaders amply proves this. They had their bitter hours of wrestling with the powers of darkness, hours which almost counter-balanced the hours of uplift. Only clearly thought-out intellectual convictions reinforced by the habit of daily righteous living can secure the soul against such emotional aberrations.

Danger of Reaction

Therefore, although the religious excitability of adolescence must not be thwarted lest it be turned into less helpful channels, and lest religion lose all the beauty and compelling power lent to it by the glow of youthful feelings, yet it must be so balanced and ordered by a clear reason, and especially by the habit of putting each enthusiasm to the test of conduct, that the young mind may remain true to its law of growth, developing harmoniously on all three sides at once.

The danger of permitting a young boy or girl while under the influence of this emotional instability to enter into any special form of religious service is the danger of reaction. He will discover that all is not as his early vision led him to suppose—because that early vision was of things too high and holy for any earthly realization—and he may turn against what seems to him to be hypocrisy and pretense with a bitterness proportioned to his former love. Many honest, faithful men and women remain in this state of reaction for the rest of their lives.

A Difficult Period

Nevertheless, it will not do to thwart these young beginnings. They must neither be nipped in the bud nor forced to a premature ripening. Above all they must not be suffered to endure the killing frost of ridicule. The period is a difficult one, but, as Dr. Stanley Hall points out, it is supremely the mother's opportunity. If she can hold her boy's or her girl's confidence now, can ease their eager young hearts with an intelligent sympathy, she can probably keep them from any public commitment. Perhaps they may desire to confide in the minister; if so, let the mother confide in him first. Perhaps they have bosom friends, passing through the same stirring experience; then let the mother win over these friends.

Her object should be to shelter this beautiful sentiment; to keep it safe from exposure; above all, to utilize it as a motive-power—as an incentive to noble action. The Kindergarten rule is a good one: as quick as a love springs in a child's breast, give it something to do. When the love of God awakes there, give it much to do. Usually, the only way open is to join the church, to make a public profession. The wise mother will see to it that there are other ways, urging the young knight to serve his King by going forth into the world immediately about him and fighting against all forms of evil, giving him a practical, definite quest. The result of such restriction of public speech, and stimulation of private deed, will be a sincere, lowly-minded religion, so inwoven with the truest activities as to be inseparable from them. Such a religion knows no reaction.

Bible Study

Now is supremely the time for a study of the Bible. Interesting as a Divine Story Book to the young children, it becomes the Book of Life to these older ones. In teaching it at home, a few simple rules need to be borne in mind. The first is that the Bible must be thought of not as a series of disconnected texts and thoughts, but as a connected whole. The division of King James' Bible into verses and chapters is but poorly adapted to this purpose. The illogical, strange character of the paragraphing, as measured by the standards of modern English, is apparent at a glance, for often a verse will end in the middle of a sentence, and the sentence be concluded in the next verse. The chapters in the same way often fail to finish the subject with which they deal, and sometimes include several subjects. Therefore, the mother who undertakes to read the Bible to her children needs first to go through the lesson herself, and to decide what subject, not what chapter, she will take up that day. There is a reader's edition of the Bible, and one called the "Children's Bible," both of which aim to leave out all repetition and references and to arrange the Bible narrative in a simple, consecutive order, nevertheless employing the beautiful Bible language. These editions might prove of considerable help to mothers who feel unequal to doing the work by themselves.

Children's Bible

Second, comparable to this in importance is the reading of the Bible and talking about it in a perfectly ordinary tone of voice; for what you want is to make the Bible teachings live in to-day. You must not, therefore, suggest by your tone or manner that they belong to another day, and that they are, in some sense, to be shut out from common life and speech. This does not mean such common use of Biblical phrases in every day conversation as to cause it to grow into that form or irreverence known as cant, but it does mean simple usage of Bible thought, and the effort to fit it to the conditions of daily life. Such a habit in itself will force any family to discriminate as to what things in the Bible are living and eternal, and what things belong rightly to that far away time and place of which the Bible narrative treats, thus practicing both teacher and pupils—that is, both parents and children—in the art of finding the universal spirit of truth under all temporal disguises. Without this art the Bible is a closed book, even to the closest student.

Making Lessons Real

Again, every effort should be made to help the home Bible class to understand the period studied in that week's lesson, and to this end secular literature and art should be freely called upon, not only such stories, for example, as "Ben Hur," but other stories not necessarily religious, which deal with the same time and place; they are of great help in putting vividly before the children and parents the temporal setting of the eternal stories. Cannon Farrar's "Life of Christ" is a very great help to the realization of the New Testament scenes, as is also Tissot's "Pictorial Life of Christ." In short every art should be made to deepen and clarify the conceptions roused by the study of the Bible.

In Conclusion

The mother who undertakes the tremendous task of rightly training her children, will need to exercise herself daily in all the Christian virtues—and if there are any Pagan ones not included under faith, hope, charity, patience, and humility, to exercise those also. With these virtues to support her, she will be able to use whatever knowledge she may acquire. Without them she can do nothing.

TEST QUESTIONS

The following questions constitute the "written recitation" which the regular members of the A.S.H.E. answer in writing and send in for the correction and comment of the instructor. They are intended to emphasize and fix in the memory the most important points in the lesson.

STUDY OF CHILD LIFE

PART III

Read Carefully. In answering these questions you are earnestly requested *not* to answer according to the text-book where opinions are asked for, but to answer according to conviction. In all cases credit will be given for thought and original observation. Place your name and full address at the head of the paper; use your own words so that your instructor may be sure that you understand the subject.

1. How can you bring the influence of art to bear upon your child?

2. What is the influence of music? How can you employ it?

3. Do you believe in fairy tales for children? State your reasons.

4. How would you encourage the love of nature in your child?

5. What is it that the Kindergarten can do better than the home?

6. Suppose that your child had some undesirable acquaintances, how would you meet the situation?

7. What can you say of accomplishments for children?

8. If manual training, physical culture, domestic science, etc., are not taught in your schools and you wish your children to get some of the advantages of these studies, how will you set about it?

9. What do you understand to be the correlation of studies?

10. Should parents become acquainted with the teachers of their children and their methods? Why?

11. How may children be taught the use of money?

12. State the advantages and disadvantages of Sunday schools. What have they meant in *your own* experience?

13. How will you train your child religiously? Can anyone take this task from you?

14. What rules must be borne in mind in teaching the Bible at home?

15. Give some experience of your own (or of a friend) in the training of a child wherein a success has been achieved.

16. Are there any questions you would like to ask or subjects which you wish to discuss in connection with the lessons on the Study of Child Life?

Note.—After completing the test sign it with your full name.

Supplementary Notes

on

STUDY OF CHILD LIFE

BY MARION FOSTER WASHBURNE

APPLICATION OF PRINCIPLES.

In this "Study of Child Life" we have considered some of the fundamental principles of education. When we think of the complex inheritance of the American people it is, perhaps, no wonder that many families contain individuals varying so widely from each other as to seem to require each a complete system of education all to himself. We are a people born late in the history of the race, and our blood is mingled of the Norseman's, the Celt's, and the Latin's. Advancing civilization alone would tend to make us more complex, our problems more subtle; but in addition to this we are mixed of all races, and born in times so strenuous that, sooner or later, every fibre of our weaving is strained and brought into prominence.

In the letters from my students this fact, with which I was already familiar in a general sort of way, has been brought more particularly to my attention. In all cases, the situation has been responsible for much confusion and difficulty. In a good many, it has led to family tragedies, varying in magnitude from the unhappiness of the misunderstood child to that of the lonely woman, suffering in adult life from the faults of her upbringing, and the failure of the family ties whose need she felt the more as the duties of motherhood pressed upon her. If it were possible for me to violate the confidence of my pupils I could prove very conclusively that the old-fashioned system of bringing up children on the three R's and a spanking did not work so well as some persons seem to think. I could prove that the problem has grown past the point where instinct and tradition may be held as sufficient to solve it. Everyone, seeing these letters, would be obliged to confess, "Yes, indeed, here is plain need of training for parents." Yet, at the same time, these same persons would be tempted to inquire, "But can any training meet such a difficult situation?"

Here is despair; and some cause for it. When one's own mother has not understood one; when one has lived lonely in the midst of brothers and sisters who are more strange than strangers; when one's childhood is full of the memory of obscure but intense sufferings, one flies for relief, perhaps, to any one who offers it hopefully enough; but one does not really expect to get it. *Can* training, especially by correspondence, meet the need?

Not wholly, of course, let us be frank to admit. No amount of theory, however excellent, can take the place of the drill given only in the hard school of experience. But when the theory is not merely theory, but sound principle, based on scientific observation, confirmed by the wide experience of many persons, it is as valuable in practical life as any rule of mathematics to the practical engineer. We all know that the technical correspondence schools really do fit young mechanics to move on and up in the trade. By correspondence he is given what Froebel calls the interpreting word. The experience in application the student has to supply himself.

So in the matter of education. There are genuine principles which underlie the development of every child that lives—even the feeble-minded, deaf, and blind. Read Helen Keller's wonderful life, if you want to see the proof of it. Just as surely as a child has two legs and has to learn to walk on them by a series of prolonged experiments, just so surely he has (a) a sense of justice, (b) an instinct for freedom, (c) a love of play. Every kind of child has all these instincts, as much as he has love for food and drink; and to educate him consists in developing these instincts into (a) the habit of dealing justly by others, (b) the right use of freedom, (c) love of work. The particular methods may differ. The principles *do not and CANNOT DIFFER*.

She who would succeed in child training must hold to these truths with all her might and main—making them, in fact, her religion, for they are the doctrines of the Christian religion as applied to motherhood. To hold them lightly, or even experimentally, will not do. One most walk in faith. And that the faith may not be blind, but may be based on experience and understanding, let me suggest this means of proof: Instead of asking yourself how the laws laid down in these little books would fit this or that particular child, your own or another's, ask how they would have fitted you, if they had been applied to you by your own mother. Take the chapter on faults, pick out the one which was yours, in childhood—oh, of course, you've got over it now!—think of some bitter trouble into which that fault hurried you, and conceive that, instead of the punishment you did receive, you had been treated as the lesson suggests—what, do you think, would have been the result? And so with the other chapters—even with that much-mooted question of companionship. Test the truth of them all by their imaginary application to the child you know best. When you can, find the principles that your own mother did employ in your education, and examine the result of what she did. Some of the principles will suddenly become luminous to you, I am sure; and some things that happened in the past receive an explanation.

Such a self-examination, to be of any value, must be rigidly honest. There is too much at stake here for you to permit any remnants of bitter feeling to influence your judgment—and you will surely be surprised to find how many bitter resentments will show that they yet have life. The past is dead, as far as your power to change it is concerned; but it lives, as a thing that you can use. Here is your own child, to be helped or hindered by what you may have endured. It will all have been worth while, if by means of it you can save him from some bruises and falls. Every bitterness will be sweetened if you can look through it and find the truth which shall serve this dearer little self who looks to you for guidance.

Then, when you have found the principles true—and not one minute before!—put them rigidly into practice. I say, not one minute before you are convinced, because it is better to hold the truth lightly in the memory as a mere interesting theory you have never had time to test, than to swallow it, half assimilated. Truth is a real and living power, once it is applied to life; and to half-use it in doubt, and fear, is to invite indigestion and consequent disgust. Take of these teachings that which you are sure is sound and right, and use it faithfully, and unremittingly. Be careful that no plea of expediency, no hurry of the moment, makes you false. If you are thus faithful in small things, one after the other, in a series fitted to your own peculiar constitution, the others will prove themselves to you; for they are coherent truths, and not one lives to itself alone, but joins hands with all the rest. Being truths, they fit all human minds—yours and mine, and those of our children, no matter how diverse we may be.

OTHER PEOPLE'S CHILDREN

Isn't it ridiculously true that, as soon as we get enlightened ourselves, we burn to enlighten the rest of the world? We do not seem to remember our own feelings during the years of darkness, and the contentment of those who remain as we were surpasses our power of comprehension. It is really comforting to my own sense of impatience and balked zeal to find how many of my pupils are dreadfully concerned about other people's children. This one's heart burns over the little boy next door who is shamefully mismanaged and who already begins to show the ill effects of his treatment. That one has a sister-in-law who refuses to listen to a word spoken in season.

Between my smiles—those comfortable smiles with which we recognize our own shortcomings—I, too, am really concerned about the sister-in-law's children. It is true that their mother ought to be taught better, and that, if she isn't, those innocent lambs are going to suffer for it. Off at this distance, without the ties of kindred to draw me too close for clear judgment, I see, though, that we have to walk very cautiously here, for fear of doing more harm than good. Better that those benighted women never heard the name of child-study, than to hear it only to greet it with rebellion and hatred. Yet to force any of our principles upon her attention when she is in a hostile mood—or to *force* them, indeed, in any mood—is to invite just this attitude.

Most of us, by the time that we are sufficiently grown up to undertake the study of child life, have outgrown the habit of plainly telling our friends to their faces just what we think of their faults; yet this is a safe and pleasant pastime beside that other of trying to tell them how to bring up their children. You stand it from me, because you have invited it, and perhaps still more because you never see me, and the personal element enters only slightly and pleasantly into our relationship. I sometimes think that students pour out their hearts to me, much as we used to talk to our girl friends in the dark. I'm very sure I should never dare to say to their faces what I write so freely on the backs of their papers!

You see, the adult, too, has his love of freedom; and while he can stand an indirect, impersonal preachment, which he may reject if he likes without apology, he will not stand the insistence of a personal appeal. I've let "Little Women" shame me into better conduct, when I was a girl, at times when no direct speech from a living soul would have brought me to anything but defiance—haven't you? We have to apply our principles to the adult world about us, well as to the child-world, and teach, when we permit ourselves to teach at all, chiefly by example, by cheerful confession of fallibility, by open-mindedness. Above all things, we have to respect the freedom of these others, about whom we are so inconveniently anxious.

It is fair, though, that the spoken word should interpret what we do. It is fair enough to tell your sister-in-law what you think and ask her judgment upon it, if you can trust yourself not to rub your own judgment in too hard. If you are unmarried, and a teacher, you will have to concede to her preposterous marital conceit a humble and inquiring attitude, and console your flustered soul by setting it to the ingenious task of teaching by means of a graduated series of artful inquiries. Don't, oh don't! seek for an outspoken victory. Be content if some day you hear her proclaim your truth as her own discovery. It never was yours, anyway, any more than it is hers or than it is mine. Be glad that, while she claims it, she at least holds it close.

If you are a mother, you are in an easier case. You can do to your own children just what she ought to do to hers, and tell about it softly, as if sure of her sympathy. If you are very sincere in your desire for the welfare of her child, you may even ask her advice about yours, and so gain the right to offer a little in exchange—say one-tenth of what she gives.

All these warnings apply to unsought advice—a dangerous thing to offer under any circumstances. Except there is a real emergency, you had better avoid it. If your nephew or little neighbor is winning along through his troubles fairly well, best keep hands off. But if you absolutely *must* interfere, guard yourself as I suggest, and remember that, even then, you will assuredly get burned, if you play long with that dangerous fire of maternal pride!

When your advice is sought, you are in a different position. Then you have a right to speak out, though if you are wise and loving you will temper that right with charity. No one can be too gentle in dealing with a soul that honestly asks for help; but one can easily be too timid. Think, under these circumstances, of yourself not at all; but put yourself as much as possible in her place; be led by her questions; and answer fearlessly from the depths of the best truth you hold. Then leave it. You can do no more. What becomes of that truth, once you have lovingly spoken it, is no more of your concern.

THE SEX QUESTION

Always convinced of the importance of this subject, convictions have deepened to the point of dismay since learning, through this school, of the many women who have suffered and who continue to suffer, both mentally and physically, because, in early girlhood, they were not taught those finer physiological facts upon which the very life of the race depends. Yet, strangely enough, these very victims find it almost impossible to give their children the knowledge necessary to save them from a similar fate. It is as if the lack of early training in themselves leaves them helpless before a situation from which they suffer but which they have never mastered.

Of course such feelings, in themselves morbid, are not to be trusted. Faced with a task like this we have only to ask ourselves not "Is it hard?" but "Is it in truth my task?" If it is, we may be sure that we shall be given strength to do it, provided only that we are sincere in our willingness to do it and do not count our feelings at all.

It is preposterous to have such feelings, in the first place. They are wholly the product of false teaching. For we have no right—as we recognize when we stop to think about it in calmness of spirit, and apart from our special difficult—to sit in scornful judgment upon any of the laws of nature. When we find ourselves in rebellion against them, what we have to do is to change the state of our minds, for change the laws we cannot. If we women could inaugurate a gigantic strike against the present method of bearing children —and I imagine that millions would join such a strike if it held out any promise of success!—we still could accomplish nothing. To fret ourselves into a frazzle over it, is to accomplish less than nothing;—it is to enter upon the pathway to destruction.

In teaching our children, then, we have first to conquer ourselves—that painful, reiterated, primal necessity, which must underlie all teaching. Having done so, we shall find our task easier than we supposed. The children's own questions will lead us; and if we simply make it a rule never to answer a question falsely no matter how far it may probe, we shall find ourselves not only enlightening but receiving enlightenment. For nothing is so sure an antidote to morbidness as the unspoiled mind of a child. He looks at the facts with such a calm, level gaze that proportions are restored to us as we follow his look.

Many of my letters show that adult women, wives and mothers, still grope for the truth that lies plain to the eyes of any simple child—the truth that there is no such thing as clean and unclean, only use and misuse. Others, through love, and the splendid revelations that it makes, have risen so far above their former misconceptions that they fear to tell a child the facts before he has experienced the love. I can imagine that in an ideal world some such reticence might be good and right—but this is far from an ideal world. We have to train our children relatively, not absolutely, in the knowledge that we do not control all their environment. I think the solution of the difficulty is to teach the facts of sex in a perfectly calm, unemotional, matter-of-fact manner, just as one teaches the laws of digestion. When knowledge of evil is thrust upon our child let us be sorry with him that those other children have never been taught, and that they are doing their bodies such sad mischief. But don't exaggerate it; don't be too shocked; don't condemn the poor little sinners, who are also victims, too severely. Charity toward wrong-doing is the best prophylactic against imitation. We never feel the lure of a sin which grieves us in another; but often the call of a sin which we too strongly condemn. Because the very strength of the condemnation rouses our imaginations, is in itself an emotion, and, since it is certainly not a loving one, must necessarily be linked with all other unloving and therefore evil emotions. As far as possible, let us keep feeling out of this subject, until such time as the true and beautiful feeling of love between husband and wife arises and uplifts it.

FATHERS

And now comes the editor of these lessons and accuses me of neglecting the fathers! Nothing in this world could be farther from my thoughts. Not only do I agree with him that "all ordinary children have fathers, and it might be well to put in a paragraph;" but I am cheerfully willing to write a whole book on the subject, provided that a mere modicum of readers can be assured me. I fairly ache to talk to fathers, having a really great ideal of them, and whenever a class of them can be induced to take up a correspondence course I shall be glad to conduct it.

Joking aside, however, I truly feel that the saddest lack many of our children have to suffer is the lack of fathers; and the saddest lack our men have to suffer is the lack of children. So little are most men awake to this subject that I am perfectly convinced that much of the prevalent "race suicide" is due to their objections to a large family, rather than to their wives'. Upon them comes the burden of support. They get few of the joys which belong to children, and nearly all of the woes. Seldom do they share the games of their offspring, or their happy times; and almost always the worst difficulties are thrust upon them for solution. Not that they often solve them! How can we expect it?

There is Edgar growing very untruthful and defiant. We have concealed all the first stages of the disease for fear of bothering poor tired papa. At last it reaches such a height that we can conceal it no longer. We fling the desperate boy at the very head of the bewildered father, and then have turns of bitter disappointment because the remedies that are applied may be so much cruder, even, than our own. Here is a boy who gets close to his father only to find the proximity very uncomfortable; and a father who becomes acquainted with his son only through the ugly revelations of his worst faults.

Not but that the fathers are somewhat to blame, too. Without urging by us, they ought, of course to take a spontaneous interest in the lives for which they are responsible. They ought to, and they often do; but the interest is sometimes ill-advised, and consequently unwelcome. There are fathers whose interest is a most inconvenient thing. When they are at home, they run everything, growl at everything, upset, as like as not, all that the mother has been trying to do during the day. I know wives who are distinctly glad to encourage their husbands in the habit of lunching down-town, so that they can have a little room for their own peculiar form of activity. And maybe we all have times of sympathizing with the woman in this familiar story: There was a man once who never left the house without a list of directions to his wife as to how she should manage things during his absence.

"Better have the children carry umbrellas this morning; it's going to rain," said he, as he went out of the door. "Be sure to put on their rubbers. And since the baby is so croupy I'd get out his winter flannels, if I were you."

"Yes, dear," said the patient wife. "Make your mind easy. I'll take just as good care of them as if they were my own children." Of course this is an extreme case.

There are other fathers whose whole idea of the parental relation seems to be indulgence. No system of discipline, however mild, can be carried out when such a man wins the children's hearts and ruins their dispositions. It is he, isn't it? (I don't quite recollect the tale) who was sent, after death, to the warm regions, there to expiate his many sins of omission. And his adoring children, who had been hauled to heaven by the main strength, let us say, of their mother, found that the only thing they could do for him was to call out celestial hose company number one and ask them to play awhile upon the overheated apartments of poor tired papa.

The truth is—sit close and let no man hear what we say!—that these fathers are much what we, the mothers, make them. If, under the mistaken idea of saving father from all the worries of the children, we hurry the youngsters off to bed before he comes home in the evening, conceal our heart-burnings over them, do our correspondence-school work in secret and solitude, meditate in the same fashion over plans for their upbringing, talk to our neighbors but never to him about the daily troubles, how can we expect any man on earth, no matter how susceptible of later angelic growth, to become a wise and devoted father? Tired or not, he is a father, not a mere breadwinner. Whether he likes it at the moment or not, it is for his soul's health for him to enter into the full life of his family, including those problems which are at the very heart of it, after his day of grinding, and very likely unloving, work at the office. Here love enters to interpret, to soften, to make all principles live. Here alone he can give himself to those gentler forms of judgment which are necessary as much to the completion of his own character as to the happiness and welfare of his wife and children. Someone has said that we wrong our friends when we ask nothing of them; and certainly it is true that we wrong our husbands when we do not demand big and splendid things of them.

That word demand troubles me a little. So many women demand—and demand terribly! But what they demand is indulgence, sympathy, interest—I think sometimes that they crave a man's utter absorption in themselves much as a man craves strong drink. It is their form of intoxication. Such demanding is not, of course, what I mean. Demand nothing for yourself, beyond simple justice. Not love, for that flies at the very sound of demand, and dies before nagging. But demand for the man himself, call upon his nobler qualities, and don't let him palm off on you his second-best. Many a man is loved and honored by his business associates whose wife and children never catch a glimpse of the finer side of him. Demand the exercise of these fine traits in the home. Demand that he be a fine man in the eyes of his children as in the eyes of his friends. Be sure that he will rise to the occasion with a splendid sense of having, now, a home that is a home, of having a wife who is wived to the man he likes best to be.

This bids fair to be—as I knew it would, if once I permitted myself to write at all on the subject—not a paragraph, but a whole essay—or perhaps, if I did not check myself, a whole volume! But after all, what I want to say is merely that as no child can be born without a father, so he cannot be properly trained without a father's daily assistance. And that, since most fathers come to the task even more untrained than the mothers, some training must be undertaken. By whom? By the mother. It is, I solemnly believe, your duty to go ahead a little on this part of the journey, find out what ought to be done, and teach, coax, induce your husband to co-operate with you in these things. No one knows better than you do that he is only a boy at heart after all—perhaps the very dearest boy of them all. This boy you have to help while yet the other children are little—but be sure that, as you teach him, so, all the time, will he teach you. Every principle laid down in this book, above all others the principle of *freedom*, will apply to him. He will take the lessons a trifle more reluctantly but more lastingly than the younger boys; and in a little while you will be envied of all your women friends because of the competency, the reliability, the contentment of your children's father.

THE UNCONSCIOUS INFLUENCE

When all is said and done, it remains true that the finest, the most subtle and penetrating influence in education is precisely that education for which no rules can be laid down. It is the silent influence of the motives which impel the persons who constantly surround us. If we examine for a little our own childhood we see at once that this is so. What are those canons of conduct by which we judge others and even occasionally ourselves? Whence came that list of *impossible* things, those things that are so closed to us that we cannot, even under great stress, of temptation, conceive ourselves as yielding to them?

There is an enlightening story of a young man, born and bred a gentleman, who, by the way of fast living falls upon poverty. In the hard pressure of his financial affairs he is about to commit suicide, when suddenly he finds, in an empty cab, a roll of bills amounting to some thousands of dollars. The circumstances are such that he knows that he can, if he will, discover the owner; or, he can, without fear of detection, keep the money himself. He makes up his mind, deliberately, to keep it, and then, almost against his will, subconsciously as it were, walks to the office of the man who lost the money and restores it to him.

Now, doubtless, in his downward career he had done many things which judged by any absolute standard of morality were quite as wrong as the keeping of that money would have been, but the fact remained that he could not do that deed. Others, yes, but not that. He was a gentleman, and gentlemen do not steal private property, whatever they may do about public property. Yet probably, in all his life he had not once been told not to steal —not one word had he been taught, openly, on the subject. No one whom he knew stole. He was never expected to steal. Stealing was a sin beyond the pale. So strong was this unconscious, *but unvarying* influence, that by it he was saved, in the hour of extreme need, from even feeling the force of a temptation that to a boy born and reared, say, in the slums, would have been overwhelming.

Now, considering such things, I take it that it behooves us, as parents, to look closely at the sort of persons that we are, clear inside of us. To examine, as if with the clear eyes of our own children, waiting to be clouded by our sophistries, the motives from which we habitually act in the small affairs of everyday life. Are we influenced by fear of what the neighbors will say? Have we one standard of courtesy for company times, and another for private moments? If so, why? Are we self-indulgent about trifles? Are we truthful in spirit as well as in letter? Do we permit ourselves to cheat the street-car and the railroad company, teaching the child at our side to sit low that he may ride for half-fare? Do we seek justice in our bargaining, or are we sharp and self-considerate? Do we practice democracy, or only talk it and wave the flag at it?

And so on with a hundred other questions as to those small repeated acts, which, springing from base motives, may put our unconscious influence with our children in the already over-weighted down-side of the scale; or met bravely and nobly, at some expense of convenience, may help to enlighten the weight of inherited evil. Sometimes I wonder how much of what we call inherited evil is the result not of heredity at all, but of this sort of unconscious education.

ANSWERS TO QUESTIONS

THE SELF-DISTRUSTFUL CHILD.

"Your question is an excellent one. The answer to it is really contained in your answer to the question about obedience. If a child obey *laws* not persons, and is steadily shown the reasonableness of what is required of him, he comes to trust those laws and to trust himself when he is conscious of obeying. But in addition to this general training, it might be well to give a self-distrustful child easy work to do—work well within his ability—then to praise him for performing it; give him something a little harder, but still within his reach, and so on, steadily calling on him for greater and greater effort, but seeing to it that the effort is not too great and that it bears visible fruit. He should never be allowed to be discouraged; and when he droops over his work, some strong, friendly help may well he given him. Sensitive, conscientious children, such as I imagine you were, are sometimes overwhelmed in this way by parents, quite unconscious of the pain they are giving by assigning tasks that are beyond the strength and courage of the young toilers.

"At the same time, much might be done by training the child's attention from *product* to *process*. You know the St. Louis Fair does not aim to show what has been done, but *how* things are done. So a child—so you—can find happiness and intellectual uplift in studying the laws at work under the simplest employment instead of counting the number of things *finished*."

COMPANY WAYS.

"A boy who is visiting us is so beset with rules and 'nagged' even by glances and nudges, that I wonder that he is not bewildered and rebellious. He seems good and pleasant and obedient (12 years old), but I keep wondering why?"

"Perhaps these were company ways inspired by an over-anxiety on his mother's part that he should appear well. Oh, I have been so tempted in this direction!—for of course people look at my children to see if they prove the truth of my teachings, and as they are vigorous, free and active youngsters, with decided characteristics they often do the most unexpected and uncomfortable things! There must be good points both in the boy himself—the boy you mention—and in his training which offset the bad effects of the 'nagging' you notice—and possibly the nagging itself may not be customary when he is at home. And perhaps the mother knows that you are a close observer of children."

THEORY BEFORE PRACTICE.

"There is only one danger in learning about the training of children in advance of their advent, and that is the danger of being too sure of ourselves—too systematic. The best training is that which is most invisible—which leaves the child most in freedom. Almost the whole duty of mothers is to provide the right environment and then just love and enjoy the child as he moves and grows in it. But to do this apparently easy thing requires so much simplicity and directness of vision and most of us are so complex and confused that considerable training and considerable effort are required to put us into the right attitude.

"For myself, soon after I took my kindergarten training, which I did with three babies creeping and playing about the schoolroom, I read George Meredith's 'Ordeal of Richard Feveril' (referred to on p. 33, Part I) and felt that that book was an excellent counter-balance, saving me, in the nick of time, from imposing any system, however perfect, upon my children. Perhaps you will enjoy reading it, too."

THE EMOTIONAL APPEAL.

"Doing right from love of parent may easily become too strong a factor and too much reliance may be placed upon it. There are few dangers in child training more real than the danger of over working the emotional appeal. You do not wish your child to form the habit of working for approval, do you?"

THE FOOD QUESTION.

"The food question can be met in less direct ways with your young baby. No food but that which is good for him need be seen. It is seldom good to have so young a child come to the family table. It is better he would have his own meals, so that he is satisfied with proper foods before the other appears. Or, if he must eat when you do, let him have a little low table to himself, spread with his own pretty little dishes and his own chair, with perhaps a doll for companion or playmate. From this level he cannot see or be tempted by the viands on the large table; yet, if his table is near your chair you can easily reach and serve him. It is a real torment to a young child to see things he must not touch or eat, and it is a perfectly unnecessary source of trouble.

"My four children ate at such a low table till the oldest was eight years old, when he was promoted to our table, and the others followed in due order."

AIR CASTLES.

"What a wonderful reader you were as a child! and certainly the books you mention were far beyond you. Yet I can not quite agree that the habit of air-castle building is pernicious. Indeed I believe in it. It needs only to be balanced by practical effort, directed towards furnishing an earthly foundation for the castle. Build, then, as high and splendid as you like, and love them so hard that you are moved to lay a few stones on the solid earth as a beginning of a more substantial structure; and some day you may wake to find some of your castles coming true. Those practical foundation stones underlying a tremendous tower of idealism have a genuine magic power. Build all you like about your baby, for instance. Think what things Mary pondered in her heart.

"No, I'm never worried about idealism except when it is contented with itself and makes but little effort at outward realization. But the fact that you are taking this course proves that you will work to realize your ideals.

"I don't think it very bad either to read to 'kill time.' Though if you go on having a family, you won't have any time to kill in a very little while. But do read on when you can, otherwise you may be shut in, first you know, to too small a world, and a mother needs to draw her own nourishment from *all* the world, past and present."

DUTY TO ONESELF.

"Yes, I should say you were distinctly precocious, and that you are almost certainly suffering from the effects of that early brilliancy. But the degree was not so great as to permanently injure you, especially if you see what is the matter, and guard against repeating the mistakes of your parents. I mean that you can now treat your own body and mind and nerves as you wish they had treated them. Pretend that you are your own little child, and deal with yourself tenderly and gently, making allowances for the early strain to which you were subjected. So few of us American women, with our alert minds, and our Puritanic consciences, have the good sense and self-control to refrain from driving ourselves; and if, as often happens, we have formed the bad habit early in life, reform is truly difficult, but not impossible. We can get the good of our disability by conscientiously driving home the principle that in order to 'love others as ourselves' we must learn to *love ourselves as we love others*. We have literally no right to be unreasonably exacting toward ourselves,—but perhaps I am taking too much upon myself by preaching outside the realm of child study."

THE MOTHER AND THE TEACHER.

"Your paper has been intensely interesting to me. I have always held that a true teacher was really a mother, though of a very large flock, just as a true mother is really a teacher, though of a very small school. The two points of view complete each other and I doubt if either mother or teacher can see truly without the other. They tell us, you know, that our two eyes, with their slight divergence of position, are necessary to make us, see things as having more than one side; and the mother and the teacher, one seeing the individual child, the other the child as the member of the race, need each other to see the child as the complex, many-sided individual he really is.

"In your school, do you manage to get the mothers to co-operate? Here, I am trying to get near my children's teachers. They try, too; but it is not altogether easy for any of us. We need some common meeting ground—

some neutral activity which we could share. If you have any suggestions, I shall be glad to have them. Of course, I visit school and the teachers visit me, and we are friendly in an arm's length sort of fashion. That is largely because they believe in corporal punishment and practice it freely and it is hard for us to look straight at each other over this disagreement."

CORPORAL PUNISHMENT.

To the Matron of a Girls' Orphan Asylum

"Now to the specific questions you ask. My answers must, of course, be based upon general principles—the special application, often so very difficult a matter, must be left to you. To begin with corporal punishment. You say you are 'personally opposed, but that your early training and the literal interpretation of Solomon's rod keep you undecided.' Surely your own comment later shows that part, at least, of the influence of your early training was *against* corporal punishment, because you saw and felt its evils in yourself. Such early training may have made you unapt in thinking of other means of discipline; but it can hardly have made you think of corporal punishment as *right*.

"And how can anyone take Solomon's rod any more literally than she does the Savior's cross? We are bid, on a higher authority than Solomon's proverbs, to take up our cross and follow Him. This we all interpret figuratively. Would you dream, for instance, of binding heavy crosses of wood upon the backs of your children because you felt yourselves so enjoined in the literal sense of the Scriptures? Why, then, take the rod literally? It is as clearly used to designate any form of orderly discipline as the cross is used to designate endurance of necessary sorrows. 'The letter killeth, but the spirit maketh alive.'

"As to your next question about quick results, I must recognize that you are in a most difficult position. For not the best conceivable intentions, nor the highest wisdom, can make the unnatural conditions you have to meet, as good as natural ones. In any asylum many purely artificial requirements must be made to meet the artificial situation. Time and space, those temporal appearances, grow to be menacing monsters, take to themselves the chief realities. Nevertheless, *so far as you are able,* you surely want to do the natural, right, unforced thing. And with each successful effort will come fresh wisdom and fresh strength for the next.

"Let me suggest, in the case you mention, of insolence, that three practical courses are open to you: one to send or lead the child quietly from the room, with the least aggressiveness possible, so as not further to excite her opposition, and to keep her apart from the rest until she is sufficiently anxious for society to be willing to make an effort to deserve it; or two, to do nothing, permitting a large and eloquent silence to accentuate the rebellious words; or three, to call for the condemnation of the child's mates. Speaking to one or two whose response you are sure of first, ask each one present for a expression of opinion. This is so severe a punishment that it ought not often to be invoked; but it is deadly sure."

STEALING.

"The question of honesty is, indeed, most difficult. I do not think it would lower the standard of morality to *assume* honesty, as the thing you expected to find, to accept almost any other explanation, to agree with the whole body of children that dishonesty was so much the fault of dreadfully poor people who had nothing unless they stole it, that it could not be their fault, who had so much—couldn't be the fault of anyone who was well brought up as they were. Emphasize, in story and side allusion, at all sorts of odd moments when no concrete desire called away the children's minds, the fact that honesty is to be expected everywhere, except among terribly unfortunate people—of course assuming that they with their good shelter and good schooling are among the fortunate ones. Then you will give each child not only plenty of everything, but things individualized, easily distinguished, and a place to put them in. I've often thought that the habit of buying things wholesale—so many dolls, all exactly alike, so many yards of calico for dresses, all exactly alike, leads, in institutions like yours, to a vague conception of private property, and even of individuality itself. If some room could be allowed for free choice—the children be allowed to buy their own calicoes, within a given price, or to choose the trimmings or style, etc. I feel sure the result would be a sturdier self-respect and a greater sense of that difference between individuals which needs emphasizing just as much as does the solidarity of individuals." * * *